Finally Me!

Thanks to Vertical Sleeve Gastrectomy

Alicia Hill-Marceau

This book is for entertainment and education purposes only. It is not intended to serve as medical treatment or medical advice. This book is not intended to diagnose or treat any medical condition. Using any of the information in this book is based on the reader's own judgement after consulting with his or her physician or other medical practitioner. The views expressed herein are not necessarily those of the publisher.

Author photo and cover photo courtesy of Photos by Colleen Gill

Book and Cover design by Prominence Publishing.
 www.prominencepublishing.com

ISBN: 978-1540399694

First Edition: November 2016

Table of Contents

Dedication

I dedicate this book to each and every pound of fat and unhappiness that got me to this place that I started. Without you and my weight gain I would never have realized that I wanted a better life for myself. Without my obesity I would never have known how amazing my world would become without you. So I dedicate this book to the Fat ME and say good riddance but now I am Finally ME!

Acknowledgements

Suzanne Doyle-Ingram of Prominence Publishing. Thank you for making my dreams of becoming an author my reality. Your excitement about my book enabled me to get it across the finish line.

Daryl Marceau (the hubby) Thank you for walking every step of the way on this journey of life together. You have shown me how to be the woman you always knew I had inside me.

Lucas Marceau (my first born son) You are the sunshine in my heart and an amazing young man in the making. Thank you for being one of my biggest cheerleaders and showing me what it is like to be proud of myself.

Reid Marceau (my baby boy, now and always) My laughter comes from your humor and quick wit. Thank you for showing me how to laugh at life and myself. And thank you for still loving snuggles as much as I do.

Robin Hill (my mom) Simply, thanks for being my Mom. I have learned so much about life from watching you. Your support has allowed me to choose the life I wanted.

Keith Hill (Dad) Thank you Dad for sharing with me the beauty you see in life everyday. Thank you for allowing your baby girl to spread her wings and soar.

Tammy Hanson (of Strands Salon) Thank you for being an amazing hairstylist and for quickly becoming one of my great friends. Your support as both have been an amazing asset on this journey. * cover photo and author photo hair courtesy of Tammy Hanson of Strands*

Kendall Hanson (first editor and long time journalist with Chek News) Thank you Kendall for being the first to read and edit my book. Your critique helped me to see even more potential in my book and in myself.

Jo Atkinson-Cornthwaite (second editor and teacher in the Nanaimo school district) Thank you for your educational skills and talent in editing my book. More than that thank you for always being so supportive of me on this journey to becoming myself.

Colleen Gill (of Shear Creations and Photos by Colleen Gill) Special thanks to my talented friend and photographer Colleen. Your photos both inside and outside of my book helped me to see who I am now. Thank you for your talent and your friendship. *Author photo and cover photo courtesy of Photos by Colleen Gill*

Dr. Bradley Amson (Victoria Bariatric Surgery and the first tool in my tool box to weight loss) Thank you Dr. Amson for giving me my life back. I am amazed by both your surgical talents as well as the tough love you give your patients. There are no words to convey my immense gratitude towards you for all that you have done for me.

My friend A (my sounding board) Thank you A for letting me ask you a million questions as I prepared for my surgery. You helped me realize that I had made the right decision in getting this surgery and now I just needed to do the work.

Maelene Norris (longtime friend and #1 cheerleader) Thank you Maelene for always being 100% in my corner no matter what. Thank you being just as excited as me in my weight loss and book writing endeavor. Your support means the world to me.

Allison MacLeod (friend and cousin) Thank you Allison for the support you have always given to me in all areas. Knowing you are there and I can count on you has made any struggles manageable.

Doug and Marg Marceau (in laws and support team) Thank you so much Mom and Dad for always supporting your son and I in all that we do in life. I truly lucked out in the in law department and am grateful to have you in my life.

To everyone else in my life that has supported me please know that I cannot thank you enough for your encouragement and support. This journey was definitely not a solo one, as I was lucky to have so many people in my corner and cheering me on along the way. I love each and every one of you. Thank you!

Introduction

My first blog written January 31, 2014, titled
"It's the beginning!"

So this is it. The beginning of my journey. The journey towards finding the real me. The me that is trapped behind all of this fat. I have lost who I am, and who I want to be. I need to peel away all these layers so I can find myself. Each step I take, each good choice I make are the things that I need to do to get me there. This is not going to be easy. It will be something that I need to work on each and every moment of the day. There are so many things that I have avoided doing or regretted not completing because of my weight. This cannot be who I am any more especially for the sake of my children and my husband and ultimately for myself. I can do this. All I have to do is walk 60 minutes a day and make good choices in eating. I have to be honest with myself and put the work in. I can do it. I am going to use this blog to share with myself and others the journey I am on, including success and failures and everything in between. One step in front of the other…

"If you change nothing, nothing will change." - Pinterest

The time has come for me to write my book, not just think about it, not just hope it will somehow write itself but actually sit down and put pen to paper and allow all my experiences, all my lessons that I have learned be shared with people who need to hear that they are not alone. I'm writing a book for myself and for people like me. People who have struggled with their weight for a long time. For people who don't want a quick fix but want to hear other people's solutions to a worldwide, sometimes lifelong, problem. This book is for people who want a different perspective from your traditional "eat well and exercise and you will lose weight and Bam you're cured." A book from someone who has struggled with weight and knows there is so much more than just "Blank + Blank = FIXED for Life."

It is not that easy. First you have to learn to be honest with yourself about the problem. Sometimes as overweight people we spend so much time making excuses and lying to everyone, including ourselves that even we have a hard time knowing what is real and what is not. I used to be one of those people that would look in the mirror and think that I looked just fine and then I would see myself in a picture and think who the hell is that/did they eat me? I lied to myself thinking that I didn't have a problem. And even the mirror fooled me because I was so convinced that everything was fine. It wasn't fine. I was over 300 pounds.

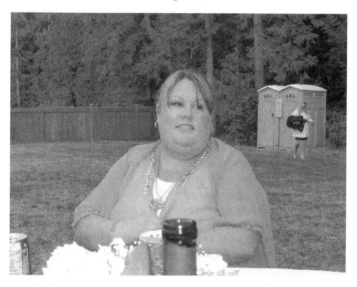

That is the size of three petite women. Not healthy on a small frame.

Secondly, you need to be clear about what you want. Will your traditional weight loss ways work for you or is surgery something you would consider? And once you have decided what you want you need to ask yourself why do you want to lose weight? And let me tell you from experience you will only keep weight off of your body if you do it for yourself and not for your family or husband or children only for yourself. And lastly, you need to do the work. It is not easy but it is possible. I am living proof of that.

My book is going to be different because of how I lost my weight. I lost my weight through a weight loss surgery called a Vertical Sleeve Gastrostomy (VSG). I am going to talk all about the process of my surgery and how I came to the decision that this was the best choice for me. I will talk about where my weight came from, and my struggles as an overweight teenager, mother and wife. I will talk about the pros and cons of the surgery itself and what life is like after the surgery. Now what is going to be different about my book is that I am going to write this book like I am talking to a friend. I will share advice and ideas and stories throughout this book, however it will not be your traditional weight loss book.

I want this book to be a conversation between friends. I want this book to help shed some light on the things that you too may struggle with. I want this book to feel like the validation you've always wanted but never gotten. I want this book to open and raw and vulnerable in a way that lets you know that you are not alone. And if this book can give you any kind of inspiration, that is success in my eyes. Let's get started with how I became overweight.

Chapter 1 - How did I get here?

Blog titled "**Was it Worth it**?" from July 28, 2014

This is a question that you ask yourself for many different reasons. You spend too much money on a new pair of shoes and then an unexpected bill comes and you are strapped for cash. Was it worth it? Someone asked you the truth about something, you bend the truth a little so as not to hurt their feelings but it comes back to bite you when they learn the truth anyway. Was it worth it? There are many scenarios in which you could ask yourself this question and this week mine was twofold. The first part of this was when there were a few opportunities for me to meet new people and get physically active and I somehow convinced myself that I could not make each opportunity. As soon as I passed on each challenge I was full of regret and asked myself why I was afraid to do such a simple thing as to go for a walk or do a boot camp all the while meeting new people? What was the fear and was it worth it? I am afraid in this instance it was not. Now I'm still slowly learning the ways of success in the weight loss field and how to handle the success responsibly and not fall into old patterns. I have joined a group of women plus two men called 'Choose to Lose". You do weekly weighing, track your food and exercise. A week had passed and it was time for my weigh in. I've eaten so well all week and was continuing to feel great. I hopped on the scale and to my surprise had lost 4.6 lbs. Wow! That's great. I was beaming. I was so proud of my success and my follow through with clean eating. These were feelings I was not used to and did not know what to do with them. So back to the old habits I go. Hey Alicia, let's celebrate. Good for you, you deserve food. Now my brain still hasn't been trained enough to say let's choose something that continues to make my body feel good but instead it says let's choose the food that got me here in the first place. So I celebrated my weight loss with food. Bad food with lots of sugar and carbs and within an hour my body hated me. It started to turn on me. My once clean, nutrient rich stomach became a landfill to horrific, greasy, sugary crap. My stomach was doing flips, my head was pounding, even my personality went from sweet, energetic, happy Mom to grumpy, depressed, pissed off chick. My body was in such pain and I could not reach the bathroom fast enough. You would have thought I drank a gallon of unclean Mexican water. If there has ever been a sign in my life this one was more clear than neon flashing lights in the dark. The sign was saying Alicia this food, your old choices are not good for you. They make you sick. It affects your personality and your emotions and your physical health. So the next time you lose weight, celebrate with something nonfood related. Instead, do something that continues to make your body feel good, like a long walk with your family or a bath reading a great book. Anything enjoyable to both your mind and your body. So the question of the day was my choice in celebratory food worth it? The answer was no. Never again.

"Watch your habits not your weight."

Have you ever been driving down the road and made it to your destination but have absolutely no idea how you got there? Almost as if you just landed there because you don't quite remember the journey itself. That is what it was like for me with my weight. I was not born a chubby baby. In fact, I was only 6 pounds. Some would call that petite. I was not a husky child. I was what you would call just above normal. The only time I really remember being fat, chubby or whatever you would call it was in grade 8. I was 13 years old. I had already gotten my period the year before and I had gotten breasts at age 11. I had the body of a woman and not a newly crowned teenager. We were in gym class and we all had to get weighed. I really didn't think too much of it until I started listening to the weights being called out. "Sally So-and-So, your weight is 87 pounds." And "John Doe, your weight is 94 pounds." And so on for both the boys' and girls' weights. They were all under 100 pounds. Then it was my turn. "Ok, Alicia hop on the scale." I swore I heard Jeopardy music playing as I waited to hear my weight. "Your weight is 125 pounds." OMG! I weighed more than the boys. I was the heaviest in the class. I was well over 100 pounds. But what I needed to remember in that moment was that I was one of the few girls in my class that has already gotten breasts and my period. And I was taller that most of the kids in my class. My size at 125 pounds was good on the frame of body that I had. I never felt that different from the kids in my class until that dreadful day. The day I heard out loud that I was different from everyone else. I felt like the rest of that year I had a scarlet # of 125 pounds imprinted on my forehead for everyone to see. As a 13-year-old girl who was very self- involved like all teenage girls, I know now that the number was a bigger deal to me than it was to anyone else. I had big boobs- boys liked that, they didn't care what the number on the scale was. I was kind with a good personality- the girls liked that, they didn't care about the size of my clothes. I worked hard in class and was helpful, the teachers liked that. So why was this number so hard for me? What I have come to realize is that we all have that moment in our youth that we try like hell to avoid. The moment that we are called out as different. All we want is to feel normal and fit in. We want to be like just like everyone else. Being anything but average or normal is always the fear of the teenager. That day in the gym was the first time I felt different. I was branded as "not average", "not normal." This is where I believe my weight struggles began.

Chapter 2 - And Then What Happened?

Blog titled "**What is in your house?**" October 8, 2015

A rickety old house, grass over grown, shingles falling off, paint barely there, car parts and garbage strewn all around. That is what some houses look like on the outside but when you walk in you see the happiest of people laughing together, working hard as a team and loving each other as the family they are. And then across the street or down the road is that gorgeous house we all wish we could have. Pristine paint job, grass green and manicured, flowers out of show room and a brand new sparkling car in the driveway. We want it. We wish it was ours. How can we get one just like it? But take a look inside and you see anger all around, no one talks they only yell. No one shares their days and has a conversation. They are quiet and have secrets. The house is a mess, the family is a mess and the inside looks and feels nothing like the outside of this neighborhood jewel. How could this be? This is what I was thinking this morning as I was outside with my dog and looked back at my home. And then I realized our homes are a lot like our bodies. Someone could look at the model type girl and think she is just as modelesque on the inside and that she is full of love and beauty. Or they could look at an overweight girl and think she is fat because she deserves it and she is a bad person. But what I have come to realize is that not all of our "houses" match up to our exterior. And this is the major reason for myself as to why I want to have surgery and bring my rickety exterior back to the neighborhood gem I know that I am on the inside. Not so that others won't judge me anymore for how I look but so that my personality and heart show up first because no one wants to go trick-or-treating at the haunted house on the hill. Just like most people don't want to get to know you if their first impression of you has judgment in it. I know for myself I have a heart of gold and I want to feel that way with a body and confidence to match. I want to be seen not only by others but also by myself and my family the way that I feel my insides look, happy, healthy, joyful, giving and present. I hope for all of us that we can all be gems of houses on the inside and outside and if we are not that we work on whatever part of us we need to work on whatever part of us we need to paint, wash, rebuild or bulldoze. This is my Thanksgiving wish for you and for myself.

"Don't dig your grave with your own knife and fork."

-English Proverb

How did I get to a 321 pound 37-year-old from a 125 pound thirteen-year-old? So what I need to do is take another look back just to see where it continued and why. As a teenager I had a few boyfriends but my first love came when I was 15 years old. He was 17 years old and we met at the drive-in theatre. It was a story you could make a movie about and then show it at the drive in theatre. However, it quickly became my real life nightmare. We were together for almost a year. He was kind and thoughtful and very romantic. He wrote me sweet poetry and drew me pictures and treated like the princess I always thought that I was. I thought that everything was perfect until he said those words that I was so afraid to hear, "I want more from you, I want us to have sex." What? I am just barely 16 years old. I am too young. I am not ready yet. And frankly, I don't want to.

Fast forward a few months and it is his 18th birthday. I have planned a surprise party for him and I am so excited to see his reaction. The shocker was that it was my reaction that took the cake. No pun intended. All of his friends and family and myself are waiting downstairs in his house where it was all set up and he walks down about to be surprised by all of his loved ones but instead he was shocked to see us there as he was hand in hand with another girl. He quickly let go, surprising both her and myself. That image had remained scorched in my head for many years, that image of blatant betrayal, staring me right in the face. She was his mistress. She was giving him what I couldn't, what I wouldn't. I rapidly realized he was not everything that I thought he was. What I had wanted him to be. He was not the Prince to my Princess. In fact, he had now become that troll that lives under the bridge. That is what I had felt then and for many years. But as I can sit and reflect now I can see he wasn't getting what he wanted so he looked somewhere else. We have both since found the True Loves of our lives and we have children of our own and we are happy. We are where we are supposed to be. We are happier apart than we ever would have been together. I have no regrets and I forgive him. And I forgive myself for the mistakes that we made in our youth.

Are you wondering why I am sharing this story? I am sharing this event because this is the time in my life that I started to use food as my comfort. I was sad, lonely, feeling betrayed and food for a second made me feel normal again. Food comforted me when nothing else could. Food quickly became the emotional crutch I used to deal with issues I was too scared to deal with on my own. Food filled in the gaping hole in my heart that I never thought that I would fill up again in my life. Sadly, food became my everything. My mother reminded me that this was also the time that I started to hide food in my bedroom and in my car. Not only was I eating for comfort but I was eating alone for comfort. This was the beginning of my 20-year addiction to food. What I have learned is that by numbing away all those feelings, life became easier for me. Nothing ever had to be hard for me again because all I had to do was stuff myself with food and all the pain and discomfort magically disappeared. That is what I thought was happening. But the reality was that I was not learning to be emotionally capable of uncomfortable feelings. My pain was actually always still with me. I carried my pain every single day in

15

the form of fat on my body, sadness in my soul, soreness in my bones and distrust of the world in my heart. I thought that food was helping me deal with all of my emotions but what it really did was superglue it all to my body and force me to carry it around with every moment of my life. It served as a reminder that these were the feelings I still need to deal with. And until I did, I could never let go of any of my weight.

Chapter 3 - New Love

Blog titled **My Journey** May 29, 2015

My last blog suggested that I most probably was going to have type two diabetes. Well guess what? I do not have type two diabetes. My specialist had called me and said "so we received your results and you actually do not have diabetes." Again another time I was in utter shock. All along I believed that I had it too. I hoped and prayed that I didn't. Actually just moments before the phone call I sent a prayer out there saying okay whatever happens if I do or do not I will work with what I am dealt. And at the very end I said okay please don't let me have it. It's amazing to me how sometimes good news is almost worse than bad news. I had expected horrible results and allowed myself to accept giving daily needles to my body but somehow when she said ok Alicia you do not have diabetes it was hard to wrap my mind around that. At first of course you're excited. You feel like you've dodged a bullet, missed that land mine and all is right with the world.

But then reality sets in. And what you had expected is no longer the truth now you have to wrap your mind around that. It's ridiculous to feel disappointed but I think I actually was. And so I asked myself why? Why am I feeling this way? And what I came up with was that I thought I had a problem and a solution, they came together in a nicely wrapped package called Type Two Diabetes. I thought that the medication would be a step closer and quicker to weight loss for me. But then the carpet was ripped out from under me and now I was just a problem with no solution. I know it is an awful way to think but sometimes we have to feel this way and realize it before we can come up with a more sensible solution.

Now onto my husband - he started his journey on January 2015, just as I had and in less than six short months he has lost over 100 pounds. I am so proud of him. He has done a great job and I mean that. He works hard and everyday he beats this thing. Every day he chooses to eat only the healthiest of foods. And every day he exercises in some way or another. And now he actually looks forward to it. What is hard about this journey for myself is the fact that he is now light years ahead of me. He is almost crossing the finish line and I am still stretching before the race. And back here it's lonely. I blame myself. I have not kept up the way he has. I haven't kicked my butt into gear with exercise the way he has. I haven't gotten rid of all the bad food out of my life the way that he has. And because of this I am at the back of the pack by myself. I want to do it with a partner but I feel like I would hold him back. Glinda the Good Witch from the Wizard of Oz says, "You've always had the power, you just didn't realize it."

So the moral of this long story is this. I, Alicia, have my own power. No one will fight this fight for me, no one will take this journey for me. I cannot expect my husband to wait for me and hold himself back on my account. I can just accept the support he has always given me. I can't expect Type Two diabetes and a needle everyday to be my solution. I can make good choices, work out and keep going be my answer. Ronda Rousey the MMA/UFC fighter has a quote that says "most people focus on the wrong thing, they focus on the results and not the process." It's true I am losing sight of the process, of learning, of becoming strong physically and mentally with each step that I take. That is my journey.

> "Darling, don't forget to fall in
> love with yourself first."

I actually survived the pain from my first heartbreak and became almost normal enough to start searching for a new love in my life. In wandered my future husband. Nothing I had ever expected. We met in college only a few short weeks after I had said to myself I am up for anything but don't need anything too serious. The universe said, "Ok nothing too serious?" We will send you the man that you will spend 20 years with (and more to come), have two children with and go through everything that life has to send your way. That's not serious, right?

It took a while for me to take down all my protective walls and actually let him fully in. He said that he loved me long before I was capable enough to say it to him. He wanted all of me. I wasn't ready to give that to him yet. He promised me on many occasions he would never hurt me the way "that guy" did. He said wouldn't it be sad if we were the best thing for one another and you never give it a chance because you are afraid? He was right. In order to move on and have a real life I had to take a chance. I had to trust him and trust myself.

Trust that I could be vulnerable and still be okay. And I did. I jumped off of the scariest ledge and took a chance on love and took a chance on him. To this day I am so glad that I did.

Chapter 4 - Our Weight Together as a Couple

Blog titled **"It Takes Two"** April 10, 2014

Good things come in pairs: a pair of shoes, a pair of earrings, a pair of hearts and a partnership. It takes two halves to make a whole in life and in relationships. This is the same for people that are on a weight loss journey. They need both people in the relationship to be on a path to good health. This is especially true if both people need to lose weight such as my husband and I. In order for us to be successful, we need to do it together. Well as you may already know this is not the case for the two of us. We are like two ships in the night, passing only for a moment but constantly going in the opposite direction. We have never in our 17 years together, been on the journey at the same time for more than a few days. One is on and the other is off. When one is up and the other is down. It is the world's worst roller coaster; you never get to enjoy the ride at the same time. And to say the least this is quite sabotaging to the other person. I will take full responsibility as the buyer, provider and maker of the food for my family. I make the meals, lunches and dinners and provide the choices in the pantry, and those who know me, know just how many times I have done the whole pantry clean out, trying to provide good choices for myself and my family. And then slowly the things that I had taken out make their way back in.

Eventually another purge is required. Needless to say this is very difficult to find or have any sort of success, when you are constantly battling temptations in front of you. Not only is this mentally exhausting it takes a toll on you both physically and emotionally too. It would be like an alcoholic living at a bar or a drug addict living in a pharmacy, temptations are all around you. I wish I knew a solution or a magic trick to get us both on this ride at the same time. Going on any journey by yourself is lonely, especially when your loved one is waiting for you at home doing that which you are trying to avoid.

Sometimes I feel like I have come so far and then all of a sudden it is like back to the drawing board trying to figure out what will work for us. I want to leave on a positive note because I feel that this is what my blog is all about - taking the hard things and turning them into something wonderful. So I will say this, I have never wanted anything more than to experience and succeed on this journey with anyone, than I want to with my husband Daryl. And I know in my heart of hearts it will happen because I won't give up.

When I met my husband Daryl I was 170 pounds and a size 14 and he was about 350 pounds. To be completely honest, at first I was uncomfortable with that. But not for the reason that you think. I was always attracted to him no matter what his weight was. It didn't matter to me what other people thought of him. I think that I was uncomfortable with his weight because I saw it as a reflection of my own insecurities. I saw how he felt "less than" when he was in public because of the looks that he would get from others. I saw he would shrink himself to make others feel bigger. I noticed that he would never look at himself in the mirror when he would pass one by when he was overweight. He didn't like his own reflection. And there were times that I would feel all those same things. I saw in him what I didn't like about myself.

Living with and loving someone who is like you or how you feel about yourself is like walking around with a mirror attached to you and constantly seeing that part of you staring back that you are trying like crazy to avoid.

Our life was not one of fairy tales. We were not the couple you would see in movies that make love on crisp white sheets in full hair and makeup. We were not that couple that would hold hands running down the beach together. We were more of that couple that spent so much time together but yet it was like we were alone. We were always eating, at a movie or watching television. We were the chill out couple and not the physically active couple. We were the getting-too-fat-to-do-anything couple. We loved one another, I know this for sure, but we had a hard time showing one another as we didn't know how to show love to ourselves.

There were times that I felt closer to Daryl than anyone else on earth, but then there were those times that our weight put so much distance between us both emotionally and physically.

We have never been able to fully wrap our arms around one another. Is that not the saddest thing ever? Two people who love one another yet they cannot get close enough to the other person to show them just how much they love them.

Our weight affected the two of us and our relationship in many ways. We were not able to be as close to one another as we wanted to be on many levels. As an overweight person you not only carry around all that extra weight but you also have huge walls put up to block any and all pain. How can two people get close with all of these blockades stopping them? We thought we were close, but we were not nearly as close as we thought as we are today. Today our walls are down, our weight is off and our arms are wrapped tightly around one another, tighter and closer than ever before.

When our weights were at their highest, our esteem was at its lowest. We would always talk about this amazing life that we wanted with one another. But this was not the life that we wanted. We had dreams and ideas and plans and the life that we have is not what we had dreamed for ourselves. It was our nightmare.

Our communication when were that fat couple was also affected by the excess weight we lugged around with us. We didn't know how to communicate with each other what we truly wanted because we didn't know ourselves. How can you ask for something when you don't know what it is that you want?

When I used to think about what I would be like as a wife, I always pictured myself with an immaculately clean home, exquisite cuisine on the table and a tigress in the bedroom. This is what I wanted for myself and for my husband. But the reality is that HEAVY does not want to cook and clean and make love, HEAVY wants to sit and relax and hope that it all takes care of itself.

Chapter 5 - Our Journeys Solo

Blog titled "**One small step**" April 3, 2014

I t really is the first step that is the hardest. But I ask myself, why? Why is it so hard that I would rather avoid it than put one foot in front of the other and go? For me this week helped me to find the answers I was looking for and it helped me to take the dreaded first step. I believe the first steps are the hardest because there is the unknown. You don't know what something feels like until you experience it, just like with exercise. In my head, for someone who has not exercised in over two years it feels like an impossible feat. I make it so much bigger than what it really is. So if I continue to think about the gravity of the exercise situation and taking the first step than I can make excuses, avoid it, rationalize my fear and simply be a stubborn old ox and say, "Nope, ain't doing it."

But then fear happens, stress happens and you have got to be strong for someone else and pull it together and before you know it you are walking over a mile in the pouring rain, carrying a way too heavy bag and it happens. You have taken the first step and you have survived and you didn't die.

When you need to be strong for someone else anything is possible. But when you critique your own strength you underestimate your ability. But fact shows, you are strong. I am strong, I can do it and I did do it, plus you can do it again. And I did twice.

So what's next? I say no looking back, that is what takes us so long to get started. We are looking in the past trying to find answers, instead of looking right in front of us. You can show the world and yourself your ability that you had this the whole time but were afraid to use it.

A friend said to me this week, "Walk with a purpose" and that purpose is to explore my surroundings, nature and get into my head some more. It is time for solitude on my walk to weight loss so I can truly find the me I have been looking for. Like they say one small step for Alicia, one giant leap for weight loss.

> "Be proud of every step you
> take towards your goal."

In our relationship, I have seen my husband thin on three different solo journeys. He would reach his heaviest and then lose most of the weight, reaching his goal in always less than a year. We would tip the scales together and then promise to start losing weight together on Monday. You know how it goes? You have your last supper and then some. You fully intend to somehow crack the code and in a short time become skinny. That is what our hope was. But it was never our reality. And we had always intended to do this together. But somehow one of us would fall off and that would give the other one the excuse to quit too. Sometimes the other person would last a little bit longer but never long enough.

Then there were times when one of the two of us would be successful (usually my husband) and in these cases it would ignite the sabotage in me. I wouldn't try to sabotage him on purpose but it did always happen. I would prepare his meals and make sure that they were always perfectly healthy and for myself I would eat unhealthy junk food. I would bring into our homes the foods that triggered his addiction to sweets. I would bring food home for myself and for my children and we would selfishly eat in front of him. My own addiction to eating unhealthy food was so much stronger than the love and respect I should have been showing my husband. Not only should I not have been bringing the food into the home and eating it in front of him and having my children eat it in front of him too, but I should have been on the journey with him.

His success and our success would have been so much greater had we done it together hand in hand. We never seemed to be able to both be on our diet at the same time for longer than a week. Either I was kicking butt at it or he was. When one of us was "on it," it wasn't long until some event would send us flying off of it. Dedication was never my strong suit if it wasn't giving me the payoff I wanted when I wanted it.

Broken promises = eroded confidence

- Tony Robbins

Chapter 6 - Sex as an Obese Person

Blog titled "The truth, the **whole truth and nothing else**" March 13, 2014

Hi, my name is Alicia and I have an addiction to food, and every moment it is a struggle. Daily, I have to remind myself that food is only my fuel and not a replacement for anything else. Food addictions are one of the hardest to break because food is something that you need to survive. So, it is a matter of choosing foods that will bring you closer to the life you want or the addiction you don't.

If I choose something sweet, then I am falling back closer to the addiction? And if I choose a banana I am getting closer to the life that is waiting for me? The choice on paper may seem simple but it is plagued with guilt, sadness, insecurity and a self-serving desire to avoid deprivation. You want to choose what is right for you and you want to make yourself feel better but when all the negatives are staring you in the face, it is easy to follow that as opposed to following the path of wellness and health. Plus, it is what you know. It is what is comfortable. Addictions of any kind numb what needs to be numbed and makes all seem right with the world. Until the dish or carton is empty and all you are left with is the guilt and those feelings are starting to come back now.

Then what? What is next? How do you move from a place of not knowing to a place where everything is clear? In those deep dark moments, I could not give you an answer that is fitting. But in those moments where my head is clear and my spirits are high I would say CHOICE is the answer. Choosing to make the right decision is just the same as choosing to make the wrong one. It is just a matter of where you are in the moment that the choice is being made. Am I in a place where I feel like making the choice for myself and my future or am I in a place where it all seems like it doesn't matter? I am trying every moment to make the right decisions and I feel like I am getting a whole lot better but there are still those times when it is not easy.

For myself, I just need to continue and make the times that I am closer to a place I am supposed to be even more. Like the saying practice makes perfect. So, I will practice, practice and practice some more.

"Your body hears everything that your mind says - stay positive."

What is the one thing in this world that almost always feels better than any kind of food? SEX! Making love with the right person can be a connection that is so incredible that no amount of food could ever reach it.

I love sex. Even as a bigger woman I still loved it. I was never shy in speaking my desires out loud to my husband. I longed for that connection to something or someone that was not an inanimate object like food was to me for a long time. My husband on the other hand did not care for it much, especially when he was feeling down on himself.

I was always the one asking for it. Sometimes, I would ask and be denied that hurt. So I would take my dolled up, shaved legs, perfumed body downstairs with my bag of chips, bowl of ice cream, chocolate bar, pop and stuff away those horrible feelings of being undesirable. I hated myself for not being what my husband wanted the way I was at the beginning of or relationship. I hated myself for stuffing my emotions instead of talking about them. And I was beginning to hate him for making me feel this way.

What I needed to realize on those sad, lonely, food gorging nights was that my husband didn't like himself at those moments. He didn't like how he felt in his own skin. He didn't like not feeling strong and confident enough to take care of business but instead he felt like a major disappointment. He didn't love himself enough to love me. That is what I wish I had known all those lonely nights. I wish I could have seen the reality of the situation instead of some sad story I made up in my head as an excuse to binge on food and feel sorry for myself.

I loved sex right up until just before my highest weight of 321 pounds in December 2014. That is when it started to feel more like a chore than a desire. It was hard both physically and emotionally for me. My husband was slowly beginning to lose his weight at this time and was feeling better about himself, as I was feeling gross and unattractive, he was feeling fit and fab. I wanted to be with him there in those moments. I wanted that connection again. I felt like we were so far apart. My body was literally pushing him away because of the size of my stomach. While he was trying to get closer with me, I was pushing him away, what a change of events. He was where I was on those lonely nights and I was where he was. I didn't love myself enough to love him. Something had to change and I hated this. I was hating myself for doing this to the both of us. Enough is enough!

Fast forward two years and what a difference; our bedroom has gone from a morgue to a three ringed circus. Wink! Wink! Now there is such a connection between the two of us - we have lost 280 pounds combined. We have come to learn how important loving ourselves is to being able to open up enough to truly love another person. So, if this is you or your situation ask yourself, what is more important, a connection to another human being or the connection you think you have to food? Do you want a food high or a love high? Do you want Oreo's or an orgasm? If you are ever feeling as I was on those sad evenings, instead of making the same mistakes that I did, turn to something better, yourself. I suggest you go for a walk and think about all the things in life that make you happy. Enjoy a nice long bubble bath. Have a conversation with someone that you have been missing, fill yourself up in ways that don't include stuffing away important feelings or emotions. Choose now and always to love yourself enough to love another person.

Chapter 7 - Just Before My Rock Bottom

Blog titled **"There has got to be more..."** April 17, 2014

I remember seeing this, "there has got to be more..." as a tag line for an upcoming Alpha Course at my church a few years ago and it really called to me. I knew that this is what I was searching for, of what I did not know. I was on the hunt for what seemed impossible to find, answers to the big why's of life. Why is this where I am in my life? Why can I not make my life different from this that does not feel right? Why? Why? Why? And the biggest of why's is Why am I fat?

There are a million ways I could answer this question but they all seem like excuses. So I will say this. I am hurting in so many ways, physically, spiritually, emotionally and more. This life as a 300-pound woman on a 5'4" body is not easy. The pain is so deep and so buried I can almost not reach it. I know because of this pain I am able to think of nothing else. I want something more, a life without this pain, a life that is for me and is healthy and happy. But I am stopped by these feelings of loneliness and sorrow. The hurt goes away when I pour out my soul on these pages, but then it comes back and it is painful and I feel sorry for myself. So sorry that I don't want to do what is necessary for my body to stop feeling this way. So then it all comes back to the why?

I haven't been walking since I wrote about it. I haven't eaten for more than a couple of days. I am not doing what is necessary and I feel like crap. I go and see my doctor in two weeks and I haven't lost any weight. I am so stuck. I want to be 100% honest and tell the world that I am struggling and I am in need of some butt kicking or some encouragement. I am not exactly sure what at this moment. All I know is that some more digging is necessary as to why I have such pain and what has caused this in my life. When I hold onto this pain I know I am holding onto the weight too. So it is time to…Let it Go!

"When I lost all of my excuses, I found my results"

How was I feeling just before my rock bottom? There are no other words to describe how I felt physically other than like an inflated balloon about to burst at any moment. My body was sore. My muscles were sore. I could barely sleep. I had such bad sleep apnea. It was to the point that life was too hard for me to enjoy regular activities such as walking or playing with my children. I truly felt like I could not put another foot in front of the other because I was so exhausted. But I did. Not only for my family and my children, but for myself, because even as low as I felt I knew someday I would be on the other side of this HELL.

How was I feeling emotionally? I was feeling invisible, especially outside of my home. I felt as if the world saw me but chose to ignore me. It is like people were looking through me. In retrospect, I now know that this was because I was hiding. They could not see me because I was too ashamed of what I had become for anyone to truly see me.

I hid myself from the world but used the excuse of people's cruelty as a reason to stay stuck. A reason I could use to eat and push away any feeling, an excuse to hide from myself. I don't know if I wanted the world to know me like this. I wasn't who I was supposed to be. I was a figment of who I should have been.

I remember one time going into a store and watching this woman walk out. She was just an average looking woman but she beamed like a megastar of happiness and radiance. I could see her personality shining through even though she never said a word. People were drawn to her. They took second glances back at her just to get a piece of whatever it was that she was exuding. It amazed me. I thought to myself this is how I want to be in the world. I want to light up a room, even though I don't say a thing.

What I learned was that people are attracted to happiness. People want to be part of whatever that is. They are drawn to positivity. And while I was feeling invisible to the world and to myself what was really going on was that I was exuding self loathing, disgust, anger and sadness. This was coming from my soul. Instead of people being drawn to that they wanted to get as far away from it as possible. Why wouldn't they? At that time, I had no happiness to give. Not only to strangers but worse than that to myself. That woman's happiness and beams of light came from the fact that she was 100% comfortable and confident in who she was, people were drawn to her love of herself. She was a woman who didn't care about the attention of others but gave that attention to herself. She wasn't dependent on whether others liked her to fill her up, to give her validation or love. She had that all on her own. I wanted this and I knew that one day I would have it. I will say today I am so very close to being where that woman was on the day I felt her sunshine pass my way. I would like to thank her for showing me what reflection I want to see in my mirror.

Chapter 8 - Myself on a Diet

Blog titled **"Why is the beginning always the hardest?"** February 10, 2014

In order for my life to start becoming what I want it to, I was told by the doctor to do two things, walk 60 minutes a day and make healthy food choices. This should not have been hard. Pretty simple. But do you think that I could do that for more than one day. Nope. Why? I ask myself this question daily. Why can I not choose the things that are going to help me on my way to a better like? Why can I not walk outside or inside for a short period of time? I have no answers. All I have is frustration, frustration at myself, frustration at my lack of motivation and anger that I am allowing this to continue to be my life.

You know what I want and what I have always only wanted? I want to have a normal life with food and exercise. A life where food is the fuel to give you the energy that you need and to sustain you until your next meal and that is it. I don't want food to be anything but that; not a way to fill the loneliness, not an answer to my problem, not a means of avoiding real life situations that need my attention, none of that.

I want to be able to wake up in the morning and put on my walking shoes and just go but I talk myself out of it or I stop myself from taking the first step. I need to stop these things. I need to make these choices daily so that they become a habit that I do and not even think about. I need to quit waiting for my husband to start, stop or succeed. I need to do it for me and only me. I need to do it forever not just for a short period of time, not for an event and not starting on the next Monday.

We have all been there with one thing or the other and the hardest part is that first step towards victory. That is all that it takes and you would think that it would be simple and yet it is one of the hardest things that I have ever had to do. There must be something that is safe in being overweight for me. There has got to be some reason why I would choose to be overweight and unhappy as opposed to healthy and full of life.

I can't do this anymore. I am tired of things that are holding me back from life and living and being happy.

I am tired of being invisible in a world of normal people.

I am tired of worrying about every single moment of the day and whether it will get me noticed or if I can still remain unseen.

I want to be seen, for crying out loud. I want to be heard. I want to bring good things to this world and to give back. I want to be happy. I can be happy. I WILL BE HAPPY. I deserve it and so do my children and my family. So, the time is now. No more excuses, no more reasons for failure and no more exit strategies ready in my back pocket. I have a life and I want to start living it. I deserve that.

> "Discipline is just choosing between what you want now and what you most."

I have spent many a Monday's on a diet. I would have my last supper the night before as my husband and I always called it. We would pig out like we were never going to have food again. Those Sunday nights that is how it felt to us, as if we were being sent to a deserted island with only carrots and quinoa.

I have been on any and all types of diets. I can remember as a girl being on the cabbage soup diet, the beet diet, the high protein, low fat, high fat, no sugar - you name it, I tried it. And at the start of every single diet I felt like it was a task too huge to ever undertake. I felt like a failure before I even began. I expected that eating Cabbage soup would make me better. I set myself up to fail regardless of what diet I was on. I was in a negative space. I didn't feel worthy of the life I so desperately craved. I did not feel good enough to choose better. I felt restricted, I felt angry and I was hungry.

As much as I was hungry for food, what I really hungered for was freedom. I wanted freedom from this addiction to food that had such a hold on me, freedom from feeling like I wasn't enough, that I wasn't skinny enough, that I didn't fit into some box of normal that was expected of me.

Acceptance from society was what I believed I wanted and needed and I thought that by dieting and becoming the "norm" that I would finally achieve that. But what I should have realized was that I needed to accept myself.

I needed to accept myself as is, flaws and all. I needed to love who I was no matter the size of my clothes or the number on the scale. I didn't need to be skinny to please society. I needed to be extraordinary to become who I truly was.

No diet on this earth can give you that. Only you hold the power to be what you have always been, truly amazing. So don't think that you need some diet to get the life you want; instead give yourself the power by choosing what is right for you. You hold the key to success. Your decisions decide your destiny. Put yourself first where you belong and choose to eat healthy food for the fuel that you need. Choose to do physical activities because your body deserves that, put yourself on that pedestal that you wanted others to and soon you will be on the top where you have always meant to be. Stop dieting and start making healthy choices!

Chapter 9 - We Learn What We Live With

Blog titled **"Motherhood"** May 8, 2014

I thought that I would write about Motherhood this week instead of weight loss. I have to start by saying Motherhood and being someone's Mom, Mommy, Mama is the world's hardest job. First of all, from the moment you become pregnant you are completely responsible for the health and well being of another person and it continues until the day that you take your last breath.

The gauntlet of emotions you go through every day is more exhausting than any Ironman or Triathlon in this world. Let us start with guilt. No matter what you do, you feel guilty, too much affection, not enough affection, too many rules, not enough rules. Every day and every decision you question is this the right one?

And even if you happen to make a little mistake in the process of the hardest job on earth, you worry how many sessions your child will need on the dreaded couch of a therapist's office, spouting off about you and how you were the world's worst Mom.

You feel guilty dropping your child off at daycare and school and even a play date because any time away from you will scar them for life. Right? Won't it? That is what you tell yourself. How about siblings? You want to add another person to your family and it sounds wonderful in theory but then when they get here you feel so guilty taking time from your first born to care for your second born. What were you thinking? Now your child feels abandoned by you. Way to go. They will resent you for life.

I could say more about guilt and how no matter the day it will always be present but let's just leave it at this... guilt is to motherhood as breathing is to living. You can't do one without the other.

How about worry and motherhood? That too starts when your child is in the womb. Am I providing enough nutrition for my child? Will they be ok? Ten fingers and ten toes and then they come out and even more worry. Will they breathe through the night? Are they eating enough? How come they aren't walking as quickly as so and so? In school you worry about teachers and if they are being nice to your babies and whether the children are bullying your child. If they are, you want to wrap them up and take them home and never let anything hurt them again. How long will the bullies' words and actions stay in their hearts? You want to take the pain away from them and carry it for yourself. Worrying and mom's are just the same as guilt and mom's... FOREVER.

Then there is the SHIELD that all Mom's possess. This is the shield that will protect her from all the fits of anger, temper tantrums, mean words, hitting and screaming and throwing. Anything that your child sends your way when they are feeling sick, angry, hurt, let down, disappointed or what have you hits the shield and the mother wraps their pain in love and sends it back to the child so they can start again.

Now I am not saying that the shield is invincible - it can only handle so much. But it does come very close. And lastly let's not forget the most important of these emotions and that is LOVE.

No other person in this world will ever love you more than your mom. They have loved you since they peed on a stick and two lines appeared. They loved you when you were in their bellies as they felt you move around inside and wondered what your little face would look like. The moment they saw you once you were born they have loved you even more and never wanted to not feel this love again. Even in the middle of the night after only four hours of sleep in two days a mother holds her child close and gets lost in the love she feels. And each day it only gets stronger and stronger. With each nightmare, scrapped knee, broken heart, a Mom's the one who loves her child like no one else can.

Even when your child has grown into an adult a mother has not yet finished loving you. It truly is never ending. So for me and every emotion that comes with being a Mom I would not change a thing. Because along with all the hard times comes the greatest gift of all. And that is having shared your heart and soul and body with your child. So please don't forget how blessed you are to have a Mom, be a Mom or know a Mom. If your Mom is no longer here, she has left you wrapped in her love and that will never change.

"Look in the mirror. That is your competition."

We learn what we live with. We learn what is shown to us by the examples that are set for us. We don't learn by being told to do one thing while the teacher is doing another. My example of food and how to use it as a tool of emotional companionship was set out for me by my mother.

My mother was a very heavy woman when I was a young girl. During those valuable educational years, I learned that food will make you happy, food will make you not cry, feelings are erased by food and that food heals any and all pain. My mother used food to express her love to her family, when we wanted and needed her words and support she provided lasagnas and cake. When we were sick or sad she always made sure to feed us full of what was missing. I don't blame my mother at all because this was the way that she was raised and all that she knew. I know she has so many regrets and wishes that she could do it all over again. I know she would make me eat more veggies and less cake if she had the chance. When you are shown a way of living and that is all that you know, then that is what you do.

So, this is what I came to do too as a wife and a mother. I provided the food instead of the feelings. I wanted to make sure you were full because then I knew that you must be happy. Doesn't that mean that I have done my job? I know that it doesn't. I needed to give more of myself. I needed to be who I am. I needed to learn that the life that I knew growing up was not what I wanted for my children or husband because it wasn't what my mother wanted for me. The cycle needed to be broken. It took a while to learn and some days I still need a refresher course. I'm not perfect but I am human.

What do you take with you when you leave the nest ill-prepared in the matters of the heart and the emotions that come with them? You make the same mistakes over and over until you get it. I knew nothing about how to communicate what I wanted and needed in a relationship with my loved ones. I had to relearn the right way. I had to learn to be honest and vulnerable and be ok with whatever the outcome may be - good or bad. I had to learn not to fill myself up with food but instead with feelings. I had to learn not to fill my loved ones up the same way.

My mother knew that this life was no longer ok for her and that she too needed a change and so she decided to have Gastric Bypass surgery when I was 10 years old. She lost a massive amount of weight. She became more confident and more of who she was meant to be. She always took pride in her appearance and stood tall when she was out in public. She was so different from the

Mom that I knew for the first 10 years of my life. I was very proud of her and still am.

Now that she looks and feels better, has her relationship she once had with food changed? I would have to say no. She still runs to food to fill spaces in her heart that scare her. She still uses food as a way of coping and not as the fuel she needs to run her body. The outside of her has changed but not the inside. She still has to learn to let food go and let the feelings flow. I know that this is scary and I trust that this is going to happen for her really soon. Maybe I might be setting an example for her. I sure hope so. I love you Mom.

Chapter 10 - My Choice to Have Surgery

Blog titled **"Learning to Walk"**
September 10, 2014

For me as a child care provider, I get a lot of inspiration from children, by watching them learn about life and the awe they have at seeing or doing something for the first time. Lately I have been watching this one little boy learn to walk. He is doing great and this certain inspiration came as I was watching him climb up a hill in my backyard. He is just learning to get his footing right and he takes a look at this hill - to this one year old which must look gigantic - and he decides even though I am new on these feet I am going to conquer this sucker. He starts at the bottom and gets a bit ahead of himself and BAM he falls. No longer than two seconds later and he is up again, this time more cautious on his journey up this mountainous hill. He falls about ten times. I am behind him the entire way making sure that he is safe, the odd time I put out my hand for him to take hold of. He graciously accepts but only until he gets his footing and he is off again. The best part of this whole story for me is the look he has once he has reached the top: **priceless**. I feel grateful to have witnessed it.

He was so proud of what he has done and so he should be. What I took away is that life and weight loss itself are a lot like learning to walk and attempting to climb a mountain. You start off slow, get your bearings and then become a bit cocky like you know it all already and Bam you fall but the trick is in the getting back up.

For myself in the last few weeks, I had felt as though I was going to slip. I talked about it. I felt like I had caught myself in time and tried again. But then life smacked me in the face and away I slid to the bottom of the hill. Not only looking how far I had fallen but how far I had to go to get to the top. It seemed insurmountable. How could I have failed again? What did I do wrong? I thought I caught it in time but what I have learned from watching the little boy conquer his mountain is that you just keep going, falling and getting back up. Look for that person or people behind you with their arms outstretched to help you and take it when you need it.

Just like the little boy. He got back up every time he fell. He didn't sit there and wonder what it looked like from the top, he saw it for himself. And his pride in doing so showed me that one day I too will stand atop of my mountain and beam with success in never giving up.

Since I have been talking about what I have learned from a child today let me conclude with my favorite movie quote. It comes from the inspiring Mater from the Cars movie. Lighting McQueen asked Mater how he learned to drive so well backwards and Mater replied, "You don't have to know where you are going, you just have to know where you have been."

> "Fall in love with taking care
> of yourself mind, body and
> spirit."

As you have read, I was not good at restrictions or diets or working or just plain doing what I was told. So, I decided that I needed to find something that would work for me. It was not an easy decision to come to but after much searching and questioning I decided that what would work for me would be to have weight loss surgery. There was a huge part of me that thought that this was cheating, taking the easy way out, not really doing the work that I should have been doing to achieve the goals that I wanted. I didn't want to have to explain myself and my choice to other people. Because I still thought at that time that other people's thoughts and opinions were more valid than my own. I know now that this was a decision that I made for me and I did not need to explain myself to anyone. I also know now that this is definitely not an easy way out. It is some of the hardest things that I have ever had to do in my life.

Having a surgery that drastically changes the inside of your body is not something that you can take lightly. Making the choice to alter your relationship with food and how you eat it and digest it takes gumption. Having 30 days where the only food you have is liquid is so difficult I did not think that I would be able to manage but somehow I did. I came out stronger than ever because even in my doubts, I did it anyway and was successful.

Every step in this choice to have weight loss surgery had to be my own, otherwise I would have failed. If I had chosen to do this for my husband, or my children or anyone other than myself I would have failed. This was the first time in my entire life that I put me first. I made my choice and nothing that anyone said or did would ever make me change my mind. I had to stand strong in this otherwise I would have failed. I was proud of this choice and now it was time to get to work. How do I go about this? Who do I talk to? Do I need a referral from my doctor? What are the steps that I can do to get to where I need to go?

Chapter 11 - Now What?

Blog titled "**Have I done it?**" March 8, 2015

I t is that time again, time to go and see if my doctor thinks that I am ready for surgery. The last time that I saw him, I was told that I needed to work harder and show an effort and make some positive changes in my life around food and health.

Since that time, it took me a little while to truly get started. As of January 1st, 2015 it has been a new year and a new me. Many new choices have been made around food and the fuel that it is for me. I have completely eliminated soda pop and in June it will be two years since I have touched a drop of the stuff. I do allow myself some type of treat on occasion so that that feeling of deprivation won't come into my head. I have heard a bunch of times that if you eat 90% healthy and

10% of what you like this becomes a good relationship to have with food. I am one of those people now and it feels great. Once upon a time I used to think that food and I had a relationship. I used to miss it when it wasn't around. I was jealous if someone had their eye on my "piece."

I liked to spend quality time snuggled up on the couch or in bed just me and my food. I used to believe that people and food equals a relationship - totally wrong and a bit crazy. I now realize that people and people equal a relationship, sometimes happy and sometimes not. This is normal living when you have a hold of food and not the other way around. I have made all these changes and I am very proud of them. I know I will never go back to my unhealthy ways because it feels too good to be right here, right now.

So the question still remains what will the doctor say? Yes? No? Maybe? Not now? Wait? I have no idea. My only hope is that he will take one look at me and see that I have done the work and the things that he asked of me. I hope that he will take a leap of faith on me and say, "Yes, she is ready and I will give her this surgery." And even if he doesn't, I will just keep working on what I am doing and get there when he thinks I am ready. The scale may only say that I have lost 30 pounds but I truly feel like I have lost hundreds because of the way that feeling gross and full and empty all at the same time made me feel.

I used to wonder how can I feel so full like I am going to burst and at the same time feeling more empty than I ever have. I realize that food was filling the void of something that I was missing and my heart was left to feel the emptiness. Now my heart feels full and my stomach feels content. I want to keep this feeling going and even if and when I get the surgery I need to continue to remind myself to keep these things in check. I know I have a long way to go and that is ok. One day at a time and I am one step closer than I was. So now we wait and see what comes next with the possibility of my surgery.

"I am working on myself, for myself, by myself."

Now that you have made this choice, you need to know what is next. First thing is to decide exactly which surgery will work the best for you. There are a few surgeries that are for weight loss so I would suggest looking into each one and the pros and cons of each. I would also say that having an idea as to which surgery will work for you going into your meeting with your doctor will help to narrow your search.

The second thing that you need to do is look into the surgeons that do the surgery that you are hoping to have and then go to your doctor and get a referral. Let me state clearly now that this is not something that happens overnight. I was under the impression that I would have everything said and done in less than a year and I was sadly mistaken. It took over 18 months before I had the surgery. There are many things that need to be done before that and each thing takes time for results to get to back to your surgeon. Especially if you have a thorough surgeon like I had.

Once you have gotten a referral from your doctor to the specialist it may take a month or so before you can even see them. And that's ok. You don't want this to happen right away because having the time will allow you to start to uncover your reasons for being overweight. This is very helpful on your road to weight loss because it shows you the patterns that got you to this place of wanting and needing to have weight loss surgery. I found this time for me very valuable and something that I believe has helped me to lose the weight that I have.

The vertical sleeve gastrostomy (V.S.G.) is only a tool to help you reach your best self and it will not work if you don't do as is required by all of your doctors and specialists. At first it seems daunting to have to go to all these different doctors and undergo all the tests but they are to help better understand your physical makeup and how your body will react and take to a surgery such as this one. I thought that the probing would never end but it soon did and then I was on the road to my new improved self. Sometimes we have to do the hard things in order to get to the good stuff.

One of the most important things that I did before my surgery was to find someone who has also had the surgery and talk with them. I had so many questions and I wanted to know everything that was going to happen to me both the good and the bad. I was lucky enough to know someone that worked with my husband and I was able to sit down with her on more than one occasion to discuss what exactly I was about to do to my body. This is extremely helpful. Knowing someone has gone through it and come out just fine will help to relieve a little bit of the worry that you may have. The first time that I sat and talked with my friend, I had a whole list of questions and the biggest one that I was worried about that I asked her more than once was, "Will I change? Will I be the same Alicia that I have always been?" Her answer scared me a little bit. She said NO. You won't be the Alicia that you have always been because that was never really you. You will become who you were always meant to be, the very best version of yourself.

When she said no I was scared. I wondered if this new Alicia is someone that I would like. Would she be someone that my husband and family and friends would like? We are always afraid of what we don't know and that is ok because it also allows the excitement of the unknown to fuel you for this amazing journey that you are about to embark on. I also asked my friend many questions about what to expect in regards to how my body will begin to change both with food and with my physical self. She was such a good person to talk to because she had just gone through it herself and was very excited to share her experience. Having that person who has been there and who understands is very valuable to you in this process and I would recommend it as a prerequisite before your surgery. If you do not know of a person locally, then I would suggest a VSG forum online. I used that as well and I found hearing the inspirational stories of others very important. It was the "if they can do it, so can I" feeing that became necessary to me. I wanted to know all the ups and downs and what to expect. I watched YouTube videos of people who had this surgery and they would come back after a few months and show their progress. They would share lots of photos of themselves so that you could see the difference for yourself. I would really encourage you to spend as much time as you can looking into everything that you need to know about the surgery and talk with someone either online or in person. Talk with doctors and make sure to ask all the things that you would like to know. They are there to help you too.

Chapter 12 - The Why?

Blog titled, **"What's Next?"** April 15, 2015

W ell my peeps, I'm going to need your help. In what, you ask? In positive thoughts, motivation and good old butt kicking when I need it. I went to see my internal medicine specialist yesterday and it seems that every time I go there I end up leaving with some sort of bad news about what I have done to my body. Because of years of being overweight and not making healthy food choices I have now got Type 2 diabetes. Yup you heard that right. I was pre-diabetic the last time I went there and even after losing weight and making much better choices in my diet I still got this damn disease. To say the least I am not happy. I am angry, not at anyone but myself. I am angry that I have played this game of Russian roulette with my body and health and all over a stupid donut or something that doesn't even taste that good right now anyway. I am angry that this is another diagnosis that I have to add to my list of all the other things that are wrong with me, sleep apnea, PCOS, anemic and now Diabetes. Come on, enough already! I got this news and I had the whole car ride home from Victoria to think about it and I came home and I told my husband and I broke down to him and I said I just feel like I am broken, like everything that I have done to myself has led to this. I am scared. I am worried. I am frustrated. There are so many things that are going through my head and I just need to figure out what is next and how to change it.

So, after I had my meltdown, well actually during too, my husband says to me. It's reversible. You have to fight. This is not going to be easy but you can do it. He said all the things that are good to hear even if you're just not ready to hear them yet. I needed a moment to collect my thoughts. And I was getting frustrated because I really wanted him to try and understand that every time I go to the doctors I am getting another list of the things that are wrong with me. I needed some empathy. Sit in my shoes for just a moment and try and understand. So I told him that. He heard me and he said something that has really helped. He said you are very good at investigating things and figuring out how to change it or make it work for you or what to do next. So that's what you need to do now. It's true. I do like to know about what I can do and what I can change to get this thing under control and or get rid of it all together. And I know when I work on gathering all the info that I need and figure out a plan I will be able to beat this sucker. I am grateful to the people I talked to yesterday, my husband, my mom and my in-laws. They all heard me and were able to be supportive. My father in law actually said to me, "Don't worry honey, we are here to help you through this." That really made my day knowing that I have people in my corner.

I am sure that it is like that for anyone that is diagnosed with something that they don't understand and know how to treat yet. They too need to hear those words of encouragement from their loved ones. Then you feel less like you are alone in this and more like you have all the support you need. So that is what I am asking from you guys too. I need to know that I am in your thoughts and that I can hear a good "get up and get going" from you when I need it. So, thank you. Thank you for listening. Thank you for being supportive and thanks for fuelling my fire to kick this Diabetes right in the face and out of my life. Love you all!

"Food is the most abused anxiety drug. Exercise is the most underutilized antidepressant."

Understanding the "WHY" behind your weight is so valuable and essential in this process. In order to know how to fix a problem, you first have to understand how it started. My doctor suggested to me to go home and write out my life story, all the good times and the bad times and then see how food fit into all parts of my life. Do you use food to cope? Do you use food to ignore? Do you use food when you are happy or sad or both? This helped me so much. I never thought about all of the moments in my life before and how food was a part of the good and bad times. I never realized how often I used food to ignore what was really going on for me.

Once you have brought this into the light and can really see it, it will help you to keep yourself more in check. Just because you may have the surgery and lose weight doesn't mean these feelings will go away. They do begin to lessen but they don't go away. It is so important to pay very close attention to what is happening to your emotions even after the surgery. I highly suggest this as a part of your process. I will say that it is also very healing having more of an understanding of how you got to this place where you are now. Having a clear understanding of the how's and why's is so important in the success of this surgery. It is like adding another tool to your toolbox into weight loss.

Chapter 13 - Use it

Blog titled **"What happens when?"** July 13, 2014

What happens when you hear those dreaded words…you may have Type 2 Diabetes, you have high blood pressure, you may have sleep apnea and it is possible you may have a thyroid issue or thyroid cancer and you if don't change your lifestyle now then within the next ten years you are a 12% higher risk of having a heart attack. Wow. Seriously? These are the words that I heard this week as I was in a specialist office in Victoria.

In normal circumstances what I would usually do is suppress the truth of the words that I just heard as plain as day, I would eat it away because so far that has done wonders for me. NOT! Then I would pretend that it wasn't the truth. Well, that didn't work for me in the past and it sure as heck won't work for me now. So, my other choice is to face it head on, the truth. I am in dire need of a new lifestyle, one that takes care of my body, one that exercises and eats right and one that doesn't take for granted that I am blessed in many ways and instead of enjoy the life I have with my family, just let life pass me by. So this is what I did. I heard what the doctor told me. I let it really sink in. I told my husband and parents and then I let it sink in some more. And then I took action. I said, "No way will this be the end of my story. No way will I go back to that doctor again in six months and have the same bad test results."

I need to make choices that will get me back to where I am happy and healthy and energetic. So, those are the words that I have said. You may ask, "What about the action?" I have been eating great all week, and I have been having a lot more energy because of the good food choices. I have been moving around a lot more. I have felt happier and more clear headed. And… I have lost 5 pounds. So, for this coming week I am adding to the healthy eating EXERCISE. And we will see what next week brings. I am proud of myself for the way that I handled this news that I have gotten this week. I feel stronger because I chose to face this head on instead of duck and cover or hide from the reality. I believe that this is the way to better self esteem, putting trust in your ability to handle whatever comes your way and knowing that you are worth it all and that feels good!

During all of the tests you are going to start learning a lot about what your weight is doing to your body. I always assumed besides being overweight that I was healthy. WRONG. I learned that I had severe sleep apnea, I was so close to becoming a Type 2 diabetic, my knees and joints were beginning to ache on a daily basis, my skin looked like I had a layer of grease on it and the list goes on and on. At first I was so angry with myself for doing this to my body. Why did I do this? How could I allow my body to fail me so much at such a young age over my addiction to food? I wasn't even 40 years old and I felt as if I were 70 years old.

The key here for me was to use this as my rock bottom. Use this knowledge that I now have about the effects that my body are going through as my beginning point to becoming successful in weight loss. My husband once shared with me a quote that I tried to remember at this low time in my life, "There is no sturdier of a foundation than rock bottom." It is the easiest place to begin something challenging when there is nowhere but up to go. Use this as not something that defeats you but as something that will only make you better. You now have the knowledge and the understanding of the effects on your body this extra weight is causing to you.

Fight! Fight for yourself and your health and happiness like you have never fought before. You deserve this. This is your time. You matter. As you are reading these words, really hear them. **You matter.** You are important. It doesn't matter what the weight is on the scale or the size on the clothing. What matters is that you are a good person, a person who more than likely puts everyone in front of yourself and you take whatever scraps are leftover. That is not ok any longer. You can't be last on your list anymore. You deserve to be front and center. When you put you first, you begin to give yourself all of the affection and attention that you used to give to others and then try and find in food. Love yourself today for the first time in a long time and you will begin to see the effects of how self love flows outward to your family as well. This is a benefit for them from you loving yourself, it is a gift that keeps on giving. Someone really should have told you and I that a long time ago.

Chapter 14 - Information

Blog titled **"Letting Go"** May 20, 2014

I n less than a month I'm going to have to let go of something huge, my parents. They are off on their new adventures in White Rock. New world, new life and no longer in the same city. I've spent 37 years of my life with them just down the road or a local call away. And soon it will be long distance and a boat ride away. I have to admit, I'm a little nervous and excited all at the same time. I am nervous because I've never known life without them here. Then excited for their new adventures and my existence as a grown daughter with parents who live out of town and who knows what that will bring.

When something like this (moving, retirement and starting over) happens in your life, you spend time thinking how life will change and what you need to let go of. For myself, I've realized I need to let go of the comfort of having my parents so close and the security of their presence. I will miss them greatly and look forward to their visits. After all, absence makes the heart grow fonder, right? I'll let you know.

There are also other ways in life that we need to learn to let go and this is especially true in weight loss. For me one of the biggest things I need to let go of are the ideas. The idea that I will always be able to eat what I want and lose weight - WRONG! I'm going to always have to be aware of what I put in my mouth for the rest of my life. The idea that I will always be fat and never be skinny, that there is failure waiting to happen. I need to reframe that positively and say, "I've been fat and here's what I have learned in order to not stay this way!" The idea that this journey would be handed to me so simply, either by surgery or quick weight loss, not so, someone up there is saying take it slow, learn lessons, learn about who you are and work towards it. And then weight-loss will come. It's not a gift or a right because who would learn anything from that? And lastly, the biggest of all is this dumb idea that I'll always be what I am and never change or grow. How very wrong. I am again setting myself up for failure. Words can be so defeating when used negatively. If that's the case maybe the opposite is true too. Positive words and thoughts will breed positive actions and reactions. If I set myself up for success with my words and actions, then it is bound to happen. So what I have come to realize is the importance of the chance that an idea or thought will lead you to either the place you want to be or the place you fear. So, choose your thoughts wisely…

There is a lot of information that you will be learning about yourself and about this surgery in preparation for what is about to happen with this new life you are being given. Learn as much as you can and be open to whatever needs to be done. I was required by my surgeon to read ten different books on the VSG surgery as well as other weight loss surgeries. I found that all the books were the same. They all talked about medical mumbo jumbo and not much about how this change would affect your life emotionally. They would talk about the side effects and all the things that you cannot do after having this surgery.

What they never seemed to talk about were all the new and exciting things that you will be able to do. I knew for myself one of the things that I wanted to do physically before anything else was to cross my legs. I have never been able to do that. I don't even remember ever doing that as a young girl but whenever I would see a woman they always crossed their legs. There was something about a woman who crossed their legs that was beautiful and confident. I wanted that more than anything and now yes I can happily cross my legs. The weight loss books did not share these simple yet very important little details in their books. There were few if any before and after pictures. I wanted to see results. I wanted to know that if I was going to do this it was going to work. I wanted to see myself as that after picture. I wanted a book that would tell me the good and the bad things that I would be able to expect if I was going to have this surgery. Not everything in the negative and then again not everything in the positive too. I wanted facts and I wanted emotions. I hope that you will be able to get both from my book.

Chapter 15 - Do the Work

Blog titled "**I am so excited**" March 12, 2015

U p by 6am and out of the house by 7am and off to pick up my Dad for the big day. Drive all the way to Victoria with only three pee stops. We are doing this. We get to the doctor's office and surprise of all surprises we must wait. It's one of the first appointments so it won't be that long right? Wrong! We wait for almost two hours to see the man, the doctor that holds my future in his hands.

Waiting rooms are always either way too hot or way too cold. They are small and over crowded with people who are waiting and anxious just like me. Waiting rooms have all different characters in them, the Chatty Kathy's, the Grumpy Gus' and the impatient patients. My Dad and I walk in and find the most comfortable seats and we of course end up by captain of all Chatty Kathy's, this time a Chatty Charlie. This gentleman talked so much for a straight hour and a half he was actually bubbling at the mouth. There was nothing we did not know about this man and his travels around the world with the Army and as a sailboat chef. You know when you are listening to someone so much and you are waiting for that one second they may actually take a breath so you can say something? You sort of feel like you are in a race waiting for the next guy to bring the Baton and he never does. You actually start to doze off a little. I know he was just lonely and enjoyed talking to someone and any other time I would have loved it. But when you are waiting for the news of your lifetime it sure makes time drag on like crazy.

They finally call my name and off to be weighed I go. I said to the nurse, "I am actually looking forward to being weighed today because I think my numbers will have gone down and not up."

The doctor comes in to see me, with my Dad and he says, "Oh, I see you've lost some weight, great, tell me what you are doing?" Proudly, I share what I have been doing. In just those few seconds I feel how he is talking to me differently, with more respect this time. That I had put in the work and not just given him excuses as to why I couldn't do it. After a lot of talking about the pros and cons of the surgery and the differences between the surgeries he said to me, "Ok, Alicia it is up to you now. You can continue losing weight on your own or you can have the surgery. This is your choice. But remember the surgery is only a tool in weight loss. It is not the solution."

I love his honesty. He tells you point blank what the truth is and so I thought about it for a millisecond and I said, "I want the surgery."

I don't know if I answered that quickly because I felt like it was the reward I wanted for my hard work, or that I was able to choose for myself and not have him say no. All I know is that it was what I was working towards and I still wanted to hold onto it. Now by the time I get the surgery, which could be a year or more from now, I may have changed my mind. But for right now I am darn happy I get to have it.

I was told that there were 30 people ahead of me on the list and it could be anywhere from 6 months to over a year. Just depends on how many surgeries he does. So, now I continue to wait and that's ok. I want to keep working on what I am doing and just getting closer and closer to my goal. I have something to keep moving forward to now, the rest of my life.

Being at his office yesterday felt great because I was moving in the right direction and I was proud of myself that he saw me as more than just another person looking for a fix but as a person putting in the work and wanting to show him I could keep doing it. I am not sure what felt better: making him proud or making myself proud. Oh heck, I say they both felt equally AWESOME!

> "I already know what giving up feels like. I want to see what happens if I don't."

Now you have done the research and you have done the tests that are required and you have begun to learn more about your body and the effects of your weight. Pay close attention to these facts.

Next step: DO THE WORK.

You now need to start taking the step towards weight loss without this surgery. Your doctor will tell you lose some weight first and show him or her that you really want this. My goal was to lose 10% of my body weight to prove to him that I really wanted this. I was doing great at first because I was so excited and I really wanted to show him that I could do it, then life happened and stress happened and I began coping the way that I always had, with food. Before I knew it that weight that I had lost I had now gained back and then some. I had to go and see my surgeon for another checkup to see if I qualified for the surgery and I had gained weight. He looked at me with disappointment in his eyes and he said to me very matter of fact, "Alicia, if you are not going to work for me then I will not work for you by doing this surgery."

He was totally right. I was expecting him to do the work and I was not willing to do anything in return. That wasn't fair to either of us. Next time I returned to see him I had lost 11% of my body weight. He was so proud. He put his hand on my shoulder and said, "I knew you could do it." I made sure to thank him for the tough love that he had given me because it was what had fueled me to lose the weight. I wanted him to be proud of me and I was proud of me too.

It was only a few short months after that that I had gotten the phone call that my surgery was now scheduled and in three months. How did that happen so fast? I was told that it could be another year on the waitlist. It happened that fast because I did the work. I could have continued to go back and forth and waste both of our time by not losing weight or only losing small amounts and not totally be into it but instead I chose to do was I was supposed to do. Now it was time to mentally prepare for this surgery. I had done a lot of the work already by learning the WHY's behind my weight, by reading all the books, by losing some weight on my own and by talking with others about what to expect.

Chapter 16 - Mentally Prepare

Blog titled **"It is a marathon, not a sprint"** February 14, 2014

These are words that I really need to live by. It is not easy changing the way that you have lived for many, many, years and thinking that changes will happen overnight. Each day it is about choices and thinking through the choices. Do I have this? Why do I need to have this? Is there a feeling that I am trying to avoid and that is why I need this? It used to be that I would make these decisions without even thinking about them. But now I have to think about everything. I do this because my previous way of living was not working for me. The more I think about it the less likely I will be to make a choice that will not be good for me. I have also realized that I am human and I will make mistakes and that I don't need to beat myself up over it. I need to just get back up and try again, with each mistake I am getting closer and closer to the new me. Especially since I will keep getting up after I fail/fall/blunder/eat/don't walk etc.

Something else that I have learned is that overweight people forget that there is more to them than just their weight. They think that they are the fat that they carry and that no one else sees them as anything but that. It is not the case. It has taken me a while to realize this but I have now. I am a woman who loves her family and friends. I am a woman who loves to take care of children and see their smiles every day. I am a girl who loves nature and animals. I am strong in many ways. I am kind and compassionate. I am not the number on the scale. I hope that more obese people can know this about themselves too. I believe that this is one of the great steps towards loving yourself and towards weight loss. I would like to end with a quote that my Dad shared with me. To fail means **First Attempt In Learning**. I know I may be attempting to learn on my journey but I will never stop learning and I will continue to get up each and every time. No matter what!

How do you mentally prepare for something this life changing? Part of what you have already done will go a long way in preparing for this surgery but there is more to it than just those few things. I believe that counseling is very important. It again is about truly understanding the why you have put on so much weight and learning how to change your habits before this surgery that will help you with even more success.

I saw a counselor and to me it was very healing. She helped me to realize that my weight was not as much of my fault that I thought it was. I had blamed myself for so long and I never thought that anyone else was to blame. She let me see that my weight issues may have started as early as in the womb. My counselor also helped to teach me to let go of blame and that I didn't need to be angry with myself or the world anymore because it was doing no one any good. She taught me to slow down and see all the good that was around me. She helped me to see the light at the end tunnel that I was heading towards. She put my mind in a space that was positive so that I could take these feeling with me into my surgery. She showed me that my life was going to be somewhat different and that would be ok because it was what I needed right now, a new life and a new way of thinking. I would highly recommend this to you to help with the mental preparation before surgery. It is another very important tool into the success of your weight loss.

Chapter 17 - Before Surgery

Blog titled **"Going up please"** July 6, 2014

I t's been quite a while since my last blog but I feel like now I've got something important to say. So, let me get started.

I started this process almost 6 months ago and I feel like I'm just getting started but on the other hand that I've come so far. In the time that I have not been blogging, I've been sulking. Life wasn't going the way I wanted it to, people said things in regards to my blog that were negative and made me feel like maybe I shouldn't do it anymore. Then I stepped back, gave myself a break from it and realized that I need it. I need the process of putting my words, thoughts and feelings out there. Not because I want all positive feedback or because I really even care about what others think about it but because it releases all that is in my head and heart that might be taking up too much room. This whole thing is for me, it's therapeutic, it's fun and it's very worthwhile for me. So naysayers be darned I'm carrying on!

Today, I would like to blog about "the beginning" yet again. So in all my "processing" time I started and stopped diets, walked a handful of times but never completed what I've started. But I've reached my breaking point. I cannot take it anymore. I cannot take the way I feel like a balloon blown up to its capacity and ready to burst at any moment. I don't like feeling like I'm out of energy before my feet even hit the floor. I don't like sitting with a chair between my husband and I at the movie theater because I feel squished if I sat right beside him. I hate the chairs at restaurants and especially weddings - it freaks me out that I could break the chair in front of the whole world just by sitting on it. I don't like that people 20 years my senior seem to have more energy than me. I hate that everything in my life is affected negatively because of food. I dislike that my body hurts from morning until night. And I know if I don't do something about it really soon, my heart won't be able to take it anymore. So that's it, this is my rock bottom. I'm not saying this as a negative thing, I think of this as my starting line. I go up from here (but not up in weight). I've learned many things down here, especially that I don't want any of these feelings anymore or ever again. There is nothing left for me in the Abyss - only wonderful things and greener pastures on the other side. It's time to get some really good use out of my walking shoes, time to eat more color in my diet and time to start becoming one with nature and with hard work. I've got to quit complaining about the life that I have and where I'm at, if I'm not willing to do the work for the life I want.

So, from now on this blog will be a progress report. You will hear of my weight losses, struggles with this and that and strides in areas all around. Lastly, I'd just like to thank those of you out there that read this and are supportive and inspired. I hope to keep doing this for much longer. Maybe not always in the weight-loss category possibly, FITNESS GURU! Who knows it's a possibility, as is life. So, now is my time to take it by the horns and ride this sucker out of the Abyss! Yeehaw!

Now comes the big one, the thirty-day liquid diet. The only thing you are allowed to have for thirty days is protein drinks, water, tea, a little bit of coffee and that's about it. I knew going into this that this would be my biggest hurdle. I thought about this from the day I learned all about what to expect in this process for the surgery. I knew this would be a huge challenge for me. I also knew that I may have a slip up or two. I decided that I needed to give myself a bit of a buffer just in case. My surgery was scheduled for November 23, 2015. I had to start my liquid diet on October 23, 2015. What I did instead was start October 11, 2015, giving myself an extra 12 days just in case. I knew I needed to make sure that I did it 100% once I reached the 30-day mark but I also knew I needed to have room to make a slip here or there.

I started and I got 7 days in and I was doing great and then all of a sudden I knew I had the buffer and I thought, "I need pizza. I want pizza." And so I had it and a few other things and I was half on it for the next couple of days. But once I reached October 23 that was it I had to do this. I even had nightmares that they would not accept me to do the surgery if I ate even a morsel of food.

And I did it. I lost 32 pounds in those 30 days. The thing that you least expect to bug you during these 30 days was *not chewing*. That had such a huge impact on me. I would sometimes just chew air to feel like I was doing something with my mouth. It was weird how much something like that would bug you. But it did and I got through it with flying colors. I highly suggest Premier Protein drinks for the 30 days. They only have

1 gram of Sugar and 30 grams of Protein. I would have 3 to 4 of those daily and I always felt full. Plus, they come premade and if you put it in the fridge it tastes like chocolate milk, can't complain about that.

Chapter 18 - Now You Are Ready

Blog titled **"Forgiveness"** March 21, 2014

This week I have been thinking about forgiveness and the role that it plays in our lives and on the journey towards weight loss. As a Christian, forgiveness is a major part of my life and it does become easier the more and more you practice it. However, when it comes to forgiving yourself I would have to say that it is one of the hardest things to do. I can forgive anyone for almost anything, except myself. Why? Why is this such a hard, emotional thing to do? Is it because if you do you let yourself off the hook for a mistake? Is it because you don't feel like you deserve it? Is it because you are still mad at yourself for it and don't want to let it go? I am still not sure what it is for me. All

I know is that I have made many mistakes and sadly I still carry them all around with me but I am beginning to realize that they are not doing me any good and I need to figure out a way to release them. So I guess I will just tell you all and maybe by doing that and getting them off my chest I will be able to really forgive myself. So, here are the things that I need to let go of:

1. Not taking care of my body the way that I should with good food and exercise

2. Breaking promises to my husband, my children, my family, my friends and myself

3. Allowing my weight to hinder great moments missed and new experiences to enjoy

4. Continuing to allow how I feel about myself determine who and what I should be in this world

5. Not walking the path I should because I feel like I don't deserve it

6. Letting myself down.

Oh wow! There they all are, in black and white. They seem a little less harmless on paper than they do in my head. To be honest feels a little better to release them and say them out loud to the public. Now it seems the only step left is to forgive myself. So for this week my challenge will be to do just that, take my experiences, use them and let it go. Can you?

You are now ready. You have done all that needs to be done prior to your surgery and it is that day you have been dreaming about since this whole thing started. Surgery day! You have prepared. You are ready and now it is just time to sit back and let other people take control in this surgery for you. They too know what they are doing. Have a positive attitude that everything will work out just right.

I remember being in the operating room just before my surgery and my surgeon put his hand on my shoulder and said, "I am going to take good care of you," and the next thing I remember I was in the recovery room. This was a great way to go in to surgery, having someone reassure you that everything will be ok and that they are going to take care of you. I could not have asked for a better moment to go under for this surgery.

Once I woke up in the recovery room, I remember looking at the clock thinking my poor husband has been waiting for me for so long and I tried so hard to focus my eyes on the clock. It was so fuzzy for me to see but I kept trying to focus on the time. Then it hit me: I have to pee. I said to one of the nurses, "I really have to pee." She told me that I couldn't get up yet and that I would need to use a pan to go to the bathroom in, right there on the bed. Well ok I was determined that I could do it. What a crazy experience that was. I tried so very hard to pee in the pan but it was not the same as sitting down on the toilet to go. After another hour or so in recovery, they moved me to my room. First thing I said to the next nurse was, "I really have to pee." She said she would go and get me a pan. I said "No thank you, I wanted to walk to the bathroom." She asked again to make sure that I was ok with getting up and walking and I said that yes I was. Only a few short hours after my surgery I managed to get up and walk on my own. This was such a good thing for me to do as it was able to start getting all the gases in my stomach to start moving around. This is so important in the recovery process to get the gases out so that you can start to feel yourself again. If you get up and moving right away it sure speeds up your healing process.

There was a man a few rooms down from me that had the surgery at the same time as I did and when I was up and walking around he was in his bed. When I left the hospital, he was still in his bed. We talked to one another a few months later and he told me that he took so long to recover and that he wished that he had moved around much sooner so that he could have began his recovery sooner. So again, I say to you, move your body right away. It is not easy. You will feel like you are just learning to walk as each step is harder than the last one but it will get easier. You just have to do it.

Chapter 19 - Attitude

Blog titled **"Strength - where does it come from?"** Feb 28, 2014

I n the past few days, I have learned a lot about inner strength and where it comes from. I used to think that it came from accomplishing goals, which it does to some degree but I truly believe that real inner strength comes from the courage to stand up for yourself when you realize that you deserve to be treated with respect. You finally can see that until you can say it out loud to another person that you believe it yourself. I think this is where my biggest weight issue has come from. Not knowing or believing that I am worth respect and deserve to be treated as such. I have the type of personality that puts everyone first and myself last. I used to think that was being generous and selfless, however I have come to realize I am giving myself LESS because I give too much. This is not good for anyone. I try and teach my children about the importance of respect but how can they hear it from someone who doesn't give herself what she is asking others to do? That is a HUGE life lesson.

I believe that true inner courage and strength comes from knowing that you are worth exactly what you expect others to give you and what you should give to yourself. I know that this is a huge step on my weight journey too because I used to think if I ate right and exercised then I would feel strength and courage. This will come, but I believe that it will come much quicker once I have got it in my mind that I am worth eating right and exercising. I am worth making good choices for. I am worth taking the time for me to give my body the fuel that it needs to keep making good choices. I am worth choosing the right foods for my body and most importantly I am worth having the life that I want for myself. I had asked someone to respect me and they did not but in that sad moment I realized I just gave myself the respect by having the courage to ask for it whether or not that person could give it to me. Today, I realize I love myself and I love that I can see it. What comes next will blow all our minds...

The attitude that you take with you into the operating room will help in the outcome as well. I remember lying there thinking to myself how grateful I was for all these people that were about to change my life. I thought of my family and how much I appreciated them helping me throughout all of this. I remember sending up a small prayer to God asking him to guide the doctor's hands in just the right way and making sure that I was going to be just fine when this was all said and done. I also remember thinking about how great my life was going to be and thinking about all my goals and the things that I wanted to do that I was never able to do before. I had the most positive attitude while I was lying there on the stretcher because I knew that attitude plays such an important role when it comes to a major surgery such as this one. I would suggest that you do the same thing too. You could say a prayer or meditate or visualize what you want for your future, any of these things are surrounding you with such positive vibes going into this surgery that only good things are bound to happen. Attitude is key to the success of this V.S.G.

Chapter 20 - Going Home

Blog titled "**I am doing it**! August 19, 2015

I have finally gotten a date for my weight loss surgery. They called a few weeks ago to tell me that on November 23 of this year I will be going in for a Vertical Sleeve Gastrostomy. What this means is that I will have 80% of my stomach removed, leaving only a banana sized sleeve shaped stomach left inside me. I will only be allowed to eat 4 oz. of food at a time and mostly protein only. I will no longer be allowed to have a drink of water during a meal. You have to drink either 1/2 hour before or after the meal, otherwise your stomach fills with fluid and not the protein that gives you the energy and keeps all your muscles intact. This is going to be a bit of a challenge to get used to. I am starting a bit here and there so it is not so much of a change come November.

When I was first told what the date of my child's birth would be, I remember having that date in my head for everything. Anything that is going on in the calendar year was always compared to being either before or after that special date. Well now I have another special date, November 23, 2015 where it will all change. My life in relation to food will never be the same. I need to become more aware of what I eat, how much I eat and when I eat. I need to make sure that what little I put in my body is going to serve me with energy and not just fill an empty emotional space. I need to become present with what is going on in my body from moment to moment and day to day. This will be challenge that I am looking forward to.

You are probably wondering how I feel about all this. Me too. There is such a gamut of emotions going on for me, from so excited for the possibilities of what's to come to more afraid than I've ever been of the pain, the surgery and the recovery process. I have been trying to get my hands on as much information as I can from people who have had the surgery and one of the common things that I am learning is that you will need to mourn food and have little food funerals to say goodbye to what relationship you had before with food. And prepare yourself for this new existence with fuel for your body, not comfort, not a friend that says nothing and lets you wallow – just fuel for your body. Those who have had the surgery have also said that even how hard it all has been and the pain and the changes they have had to go through, they would never change a thing because of where they are now. So that is what I will hold onto. There have also been things written about "What I wish I knew before surgery" and this has been really helpful. Two of my favorite things I've heard are:

1. Do not compare your progress or weight loss with anyone else. This is so true because if you do then you will either feel like you are failing or that you are the champ. Either of which is not helpful.

2. Make sure to work on any emotional issues before and during the surgery because they will still be there even 100 pounds lighter.

This too is great advice. I'm looking into a counsellor as we speak actually. I don't want to carry any extra weight with me on this journey; I want to shed the weight and any extra unwanted emotions that come with it. I will not be held back.

When you look up my surgery (V.S.G.) it shows tons of before and after pictures of the people who have had the procedure done. The differences are so crazy, like two completely different people. I love looking at the after picture and imagining what I want mine to look like. This really helps to start thinking about your goals, not just the hard start to this journey but what your finish line will look like to you.

My goal for my end weight is to be 150 pounds or lighter with greatly defined muscles. Not beasty but BEAUTY! My goal outfit is a nice pair of slacks with a crisp white shirt tucked in and a belt that you can see. Those two goals mean a lot to me but not as much as the goal of how I want to feel. I don't know if I have ever been 100% confident in my entire life. That is the feeling goal I want for myself. To not have one shred of insecurity at all. I want to feel happy, healthy and proud with a smile that lights up an entire room. This is what I see for my end goal. I cannot wait to show the accomplished goal to you, the world and myself!!!!

What is next? You have now gone home after a short recovery at the hospital. The first thing that you will notice is that anything that you have in your stomach, liquid wise, (as that is all that you are allowed right now) feels like you just ate an entire smorgasbord on your own. It was so weird that one small drink of tea or broth felt so filling to my stomach. It will get better after a while. It is tight and swollen right now and that is a good thing because this is where weight loss happens. Small sips are very important. We still think that we can chug the way we used to but we really can't do that anymore. You will be sent home with a list of the things that you can and cannot eat as well as when you can start transitioning into real food. Make sure to take time, listen to your body. You may not be ready when the list says that you are and then again you may feel ready even sooner. I would not suggest pushing the limits on that side of it though because you will pay for it physically. I tried to always make sure to pay very close attention to what my body was saying to me. I listened when it would feel tight and then I realized ok that was too much - time to slow down.

You will soon become very in tuned to what is going on for your body. This is very important as it is one of the biggest keys.

Chapter 21 - Changes

Blog titled **"What my weight represents for me"** March 7, 2014

My doctor asked me to read quite a few books on weight loss and health. One of the books had this great question in it that I have been thinking about for a while and I think I have finally come up the answer. The question was, "What does your weight represent for you?"

Now I could answer that my weight represents bad food choices and lack of exercise, I'd rather have caramel than carrots, I'd rather sit than walk and I choose TV over cardio. But I believe those are just my habits. Not good ones but habits none the less. As for what I truly believe the question means is what emotional pain was my heart suffering that I had to protect or avoid it with food. I believe that it did start at first as a habit and turned into a way of comfort for me.

I remember my husband Daryl losing a large amount of weight just before our wedding. He was all about running and salads and I was not ready to join him on that journey yet. I clearly remember saying to him just weeks before the wedding, "I feel so alone. We used to share food and movies and now you are about health and I don't feel like I fit into this new life and I feel so lonely." After our wedding when the pictures came back my husband looked fantastic and I looked FAT. And as we all know the first few years of marriage are not easy. So what I had learned before our marriage was that food feels better than being alone. Food feels better than fighting. Food feels better than any negative emotions until one day food feels like CRAP.

Food was affecting so much of my life, my relationships, my marriage and the worst part my ability to have children. Because I was overweight I developed PCOS (Poly Cystic Ovarian Syndrome) which affects your fertility. So, we struggled for five long years to have a child. And with that type of struggle and all the emotions comes eating with my dear trusted friend FOOD. I could go on about how food was more a part of my life than anything else but what I would instead like to say is I believe for myself it has represented loneliness, lack of good communication with my loved ones and a way of life that I couldn't quit. My weight represents too many years and moments I have missed out on because I was too wrapped up in my own sadness to ever be truly happy. Wow. That is huge. It is a big realization of what I don't want my life to be like anymore. I want to enjoy every little moment of each day with my family and friends. I'm looking forward to finally living a joyful life full of love and happiness that I have been missing out on. And in two days I have already lost 5 pounds. Not a bad start...

I am working on myself, for myself, by myself

One of the most difficult things that you are going to have to get used to is the fact that you will no longer be able to drink and eat at the same time. The why behind this is because your stomach is so small now that if you drink and eat you will start to stretch it. So you must decide what you want first, a drink or food. But you can't have both. This takes a bit of time to get used to. Especially when you are having something that needs to be washed down, you really want that drink. I have tried to have just a little swish of something on a few occasions and boy did I regret that. It physically hurts to have too much food and drink in your stomach at one time. You may get frustrated with this but if you think about it this way that it is really a blessing that will make a huge difference. Your body is now asking that you pay attention and if you do you will be successful.

When it comes to the scale I say do what works for you. Some people like to weigh themselves every day and others like to weigh themselves once in a while. You do what works the best for you. I like to weigh myself more frequently but then I found that I was not getting the results that I wanted because the weight was not falling off as quickly as I had hoped that it would. So what I do now is go by the feeling of my clothes and how I feel physically versus that number that is on the scale. Try not to compare how other people lose their weight with how you lose yours. It doesn't matter. We are all different and we will all lose the way that we are supposed to lose. If we compare ourselves, we will begin to always feel like we are not good enough. We need to focus on ourselves and our own success not others. Remember we are at the top of our lists now.

My favorite thing to do now is go through my clothes every few months and try them on and see what I need to throw out now because everything is getting too big on me. This is important to do because it shows you how well you are doing. You can see that you are losing weight because the clothes are now falling off you that once used to be tight. You will probably know someone who could use your clothes so I would say to give them away. If you keep them that is just saying that you have a place to go back to. Not a good idea. You don't want that. This is not who you are anymore. Giving the clothes away to another person feels good too. They will appreciate it. And you will like knowing that you are ridding yourself of things that describe who you used to be.

One final thing that I would like to share about what I have learned and what you may or may not go through on this journey is getting compliments. Before, when someone would complement me I would always feel uncomfortable and then change the subject really quickly. It was something that was so foreign to me that I did not know how to handle it. Instead of graciously accepting the compliment and listening to what they were saying to me I would get all flabbergasted and feel weird. You are going to start getting compliments now because you are starting to become who you were always meant to be and people are noticing that. It is a wonderful thing. Accept the compliments with a smile and a thank you. Hear the words that they are saying to you and appreciate that people are finally noticing the good in you. This is a wonderful time. When you start to hear these things about yourself from others you will begin to truly believe them yourself. These compliments are helping to heal the wounds that you have carried around with you for much too long. Be grateful and say thank you.

Chapter 22 - Does Your Personality Change When You Have Had VSG Surgery?

Blog titled **"Who I was, who I am and who I want to be"** March 27, 2014

At some time or another in your life you will ask yourself these questions, maybe not in this order or all at once, but you will. As for me and my weight loss journey it is important to try and work through my "head junk" so that I can be more clear minded when it comes to making good choices for my body. I will start with who I was. Who I was, was not a person that I am very proud of, or would ever want to be again. I will say that I did learn some lessons from that girl. I was one of those people that would tell everyone that I was a people pleaser but I was actually just selfish. My way or the highway as the saying goes. One of my worst "who I used to be moments" was when I had convinced my then friends, that a good idea would be to let us sit in a circle and tell everyone about their flaws. Not a good idea especially when there was no plan to talk them through, mend them or give suggestions to an alternative. Nope just sit in what's wrong with you and what others think is wrong with you and then carry on with your day. BAD IDEA! I don't know what I was thinking. Needless to say many of those friends are no longer my friends today and I don't blame them. They probably all feared that the "flaw circle" may rear its ugly head. So as you could understand that girl was absolutely not who I wanted to remain the rest of my days. TIME FOR CHANGE!

Today, that sad, helpless girl is far from who I am. Today I am getting so close to who I want to be. I am stronger and more self aware because after all the only flaws you could ever fix are your own. So, I focus solely on myself, with the exception of my children and trying to show them how to be aware of their own selves in this world and not worry about others. I have a faith that has taken me higher in life than I ever imagined for myself with even more to come. I love without any expectation in return. I share with my whole heart, both of myself and of my world. I want each day to grow to be even more of who I want to be. TIME FOR CHANGE!

Who I want to be is courageous, strong, loving and lovable, helpful, honest, intelligent with a continued zest for more learning. I want to be happy with who I am but still have the desire to grow and be better. I want my world to revolve around not what I look like but who I am and what I bring to this life. I want to be honest to myself and for myself but not too honest that I hurt someone else. I want to continue to grow in my Faith and come even closer to the Heaven on earth I already feel. I want my "Fruits of my Spirit" to shine through and be Christ-like in all I do. This is who I want to be and who I will be. Far from a girl with her measuring stick of others shortcomings and no self reflection. Bye, Bye sad lonely girl - thanks for the lesson of who to never be again and Hello to a world of possibilities...

Now that I have had my surgery and lost over 100 pounds, how has my personality changed? I would say that yes my personality has changed but for the better. I am nothing like I used to be. I was always nice and kind but I was never really happy. I was overly nice to please everyone because if I was kind they wouldn't notice that I was fat and that I didn't really like who I was. Now, I am still nice and kind but to myself first so that I can be my very best self for others. I value who I am now and what I bring to the table and to my relationships. I can stand tall and confident in knowing that I love myself and that I am very proud of who I am becoming. It is not just the weight loss that allows me to feel all these wonderful things. It is ridding myself off all of those negative feelings that used to surround me and the food that I held so closely to myself. Now that I have let go of the hold I used to have, I've opened my heart and myself up to so much more. It is kind of like the world I was living in was on pause as I moved through it not really enjoying what was going on around me. And now that life is on play I get to be a part of it all and have fun like the rest of the world. I think that my biggest personality change comes from the fact that I am living life fully now and that it makes you happy. Could you ask for anything much better than that?

Chapter 23 - Where Do I Put My Feelings Now?

Blog titled "No more what is next with food but instead what is next in life and adventure" Jul 18, 2014

A little while ago someone dear to me said, "Alicia, I wish you could see yourself the way I see you." She also went onto to say, "You also need to take more chances in life by meeting new people and having adventures!" Those things have been ringing in my ears lately. I have gotten all the bad food out of my system and I'm more clear headed. I really appreciate those words and who they came from. For myself, life is always an adventure every day. Between child care as my profession, two very go, go, go boys and a young at heart husband, it is an adventure. I'm starting to also see what she meant when she said how I see you because when you have a clear mind, you are happier and more positive. So, I do see myself in a brighter light, one that reflects who I am and not just what I look like.

And as for meeting new people this too comes when you feel positive about life and positive about who you are and the desire to share both with new people. Sometimes it's safer to stay within the same circle of friends; however, when you don't spread your wings to new people and opportunities you miss out on possible personal growth, as well as meeting people who may be just what you need in your life. I've spent too long being safe and not enough time saying, "What's the next new adventure buddy?" So this week my goal will be to introduce myself to someone new. I'm going to be vulnerable by letting myself do something outside of my normal comfort zone. I will be spreading my wings for sure.

This week's progress is I'm down another 4 pounds. Clothes are feeling more comfortable on, seats aren't as tight, and the steering wheel in the car is more comfortable. My mindset is incredibly happy and positive. Food choices have been easier to make. I've walked three times this week all for more than 30 minutes. Next week will be four times. It's all getting better and better. So new challenges, continuing in the right direction with food and health, meet one new person this week and try something new. Let the adventures begin!

There are so many wonderful things about the VSG surgery and I could go on and on for days but the one thing that is still hard to try and understand for me is where do I put my feelings now that I can no longer put them into food or stuff them into non-existence for the moment? What used to be a place where I felt safe and protected by disregarding any and all feelings has now become a vast abyss of never ending emotions, each one of them more real than the ones before each of them requiring more and more attention from me, their owner. So many years of my life were spent sending feelings away to be dealt with at a later date. And now they are all returning saying, "Remember me? You can no longer pretend that I don't exist, it is time to deal with me so that you can move onto my brothers and sisters." And then fear sets in as I don't know how to really handle, feel or deal with feelings. I never have. I have eaten them away. I have stuffed them down. I have pretended that they are not all up in my face.

Feelings are scary especially those you have never dealt with before. You don't know what the outcome will be.

It is all unknown. But instead of never being able to experience the good, bad, scary or exciting feelings, we need to open ourselves up and take that first step towards something new. Instead of thinking, "Where do I put my feelings now?" (which actually means, "Where do I hide or ignore my feelings?") I should be thinking, "How many new feelings can I experience daily?" Not owning my emotions but instead hiding them is my biggest contributor to my weight gain. This is not how I want to live any longer. Just because we think if we ignore something long enough it will eventually disappear, doesn't mean that those feelings aren't still there. It is like a child covering his eyes and saying you can't see me. Yes, we can. Just because we try to cover up the feelings doesn't mean they are still right there in front of us. We see you, we know that you are there. And now we are ready to experience you: the good, the bad and even the ugly. That is what life is all about, living and feeling.

Chapter 24 - Has My Relationship With Food Changed?

Blog titled **"It is not Just weight loss"**
March 28, 2016

Every day I continue to learn more about myself on this journey towards my authentic self. As I shed the old me and become closer to who I am, I see the world differently and more importantly I see who I am in the world differently. I, as an overweight woman, didn't want to say or do anything wrong. My opinion didn't matter as I already had so much to make up for that adding an opinion to the mix would have just thrown me over the edge. I tried to people please, even at my own expense. I never wanted to a burden to anyone else - even strangers. Now as I think back to that I ask myself why? Why was someone else more important than me? Why was someone else's happiness more important than my own? And I can see that it is about worth. I felt that my worth was less than anyone else's and it was tied strictly to my weight. It seems so backwards now that I think of it. The size of a person shouldn't determine the heart of the person but sadly it does. And it is not just how the world values overweight people but how an overweight person values themselves in the world. My father said to me recently, "You've put your life on a shelf for so long. I am happy to see that you have finally taken it down and are enjoying life now."

It was the truth. I would just put one foot in front of the other and did the motions of living but never really lived the way I should have been. I never appreciated the life that I had because I was always thinking of the life I wanted. And now that life is finally here. I am back to a life where I get to enjoy every moment. A life where my opinions are just as important as anyone else. A life where I am just as valuable as anyone else. And a life where I am not only putting one foot in front of the other but that I am enjoying each step that I take. My weight held me back in so many ways. It held me back physically of course but it also held me back mentally and emotionally. It was as though I was on autopilot like a computer running my life but not me.

As I shed more and more weight, I am becoming my own pilot and my life and every move I make is as my own Captain. I am so grateful each and every day. I want to shout it from the rooftops and share it with the world. I want people who are struggling to know it gets better and it doesn't have to be so hard. I want the world to enjoy life just as much as I do. I want the world to be just as happy as I am.

I would like to now share a weight loss update. Since my highest weight in December 2014 I am down 112 pounds. Since just before my liquid diet for the surgery I am down 82 pounds and since the day of surgery I am down 50 pounds in four and 1/2 months. I know it is just weight loss but for me it is so much more. For me, with each pound lost there is also sadness lost, worthlessness lost, anger lost, frustration lost, guilt lost, embarrassment lost, and the uncomfortable feeling is lost. And with each thing that I lose I also gain something back. When sadness is lost, HAPPINESS is gained. When worthlessness is lost, VALUE is gained. When anger is lost, FORGIVENESS is gained. When frustration is lost, CALM is gained. When guilt is lost, INNOCENCE is gained. When embarrassment is lost,

PRIDE AND CONFIDENCE are gained. And when that uncomfortable feeling is lost, COMFORT is gained. It may only be numbers on the scale but for me it is becoming the person I was always meant to be.

Has my relationship with food changed since having VSG weight loss surgery? This is a question I ask myself daily. In some ways the relationship that I have with food is completely different and then on the other hand it is exactly the same. Today for instance was one of those times that it was so much the same that it scared me. I am lucky enough to still enjoy the things that I loved such as pizza but now only in the tiniest of portions. What I used to inhale was an entire medium on my own and now I can only have one small piece. This I am so grateful for. There is no binging when you have a small stomach. Our family now shares a large pizza and I still get to enjoy one piece with the family and a piece to enjoy for my lunch the next day. Last night I ate my one piece and I was looking forward to enjoying my additional piece for lunch today. However, the food Gods had other plans. My youngest son decided he should have my leftover piece instead of me, its rightful owner of said piece of cheesy heavenly goodness. When I opened the fridge at lunch, with my mouth watering, anticipating the scrumptious piece of gooey carbs I was about to enjoy, there was nothing there. I scanned the entire fridge looking for the pizza and nothing. It was time to investigate. Who stole my deliciousness? And more importantly - why? You would have thought that I was searching the globe for a cure to some rare disease my child was suffering from. And then he said it. "Mom, I ate your pizza." Why? Why? Why? I was so angry. I was looking forward to that all morning knowing that I could enjoy that pizza again. I was angrier than I should have been. It was only pizza. I could have it again another time. What is the big deal? That was the question I really needed to pay attention to was my frustration. What was my connection to that pizza that had me in a knot? Was it the fact that it was stolen from me and I felt betrayed? Was it that the pizza meant more to me than the feelings of my son who felt awful for eating my pizza? I am not quite sure either way but the point is that it was only pizza which is very replaceable but not the relationship that I have with my son. He trusts me to show him what a responsible adult is supposed to behave like when confronted with a situation that happens to frustrate them. He doesn't expect or want me to behave like an unreasonable child throwing a hissy fit.

So after a little bit of sulking, complaining and self realization I have concluded that in this instance pizza loses and I have gained, not pounds but some awareness around where the importance of food lies in my life. Not at the front where it once was but far, far behind the things of importance like an old discarded pizza box.

Chapter 25 - Eye Contact

Blog titled **"It is a whole new world"**
June 12, 2016

I cannot believe that only a few short months ago I was over 300 pounds, sore everywhere and faking life. And now I just completed my first ever 5km Foam Fest Run. Who would have thought it? Not me. Definitely not me! What an amazing experience I had today at the run. I was becoming more and more nervous as the day was getting closer. I had never done anything like this before. I was always the one cheering from the sideline. I wasn't the one in there doing it with everyone else. I was so nervous and scared that I tried to convince myself that I could not do it. How would I know if I could do it or I could not do it unless I got out there and I tried? I had to tell myself that I was no longer the woman who was over 300 pounds. I was now the woman that tried new things and got out there and did it with everyone else. I was capable and I was most importantly now willing. I was willing to step outside of my comfort zone. I was willing to get down and dirty with the rest of them.

I was excited to do my first adventurous run with my husband. We got to share this experience together. I got to show him that I could do things like this now and I could enjoy them. I will say that there were some things that I was worried to try, like the climbing the big nets and walking on the foam in the water. So, those things I passed on, this time. I told myself as I watched others, next year I will do all of them. And I will. The scariest part of trying something new is the fear of failing at it. Once you get over the scary part and push through, all the fear goes away and what comes next is pride. You are proud of yourself for doing it even though you were scared and did it anyway. And I did it and now I am so proud of myself. I got to show my husband and my children that I am proud for facing my fears and doing it! Next year the whole family gets to do this together and I can't wait!

"Discipline is just choosing
between what you want now
and what you want most"

I wonder when I will get used to how different my world is? One of the biggest differences for me now is the fact that I actually look people in the eyes and have the eye contact returned. The confidence that I have now allows me to give someone my full undivided attention and look them straight in the eyes without the fear of judgment that I used to hide from.

If you have ever seen the movie The Color Purple, there is a scene in the movie where Whoopi Goldberg's character is sitting on the bed and she is smiling and laughing and then all of a sudden she realized that she was smiling and covers her mouth. She was embarrassed. She was ashamed of her smile because it was not perfect and she was told by others that she was ugly. So, she hid herself. I could relate so much to that scene because I too felt ashamed of my body and sadly of myself. I didn't want to smile and show myself to the world because I was so afraid of what someone else's reaction to me was going to be.

As I look around now, I still try and pay close attention to overweight people and see if I can relate to that old part of myself and the truth of it is I can't anymore. What I do notice is that people that are obese, heavy, fat or whatever you want to call it, spend most of their time hiding, hiding who they really are, hiding the food that they eat, hiding for fear of other people's reactions or opinions of them.

That's how I used to feel too. I never wanted to be me. I didn't feel like I was good enough for the world. Our worth should never be based on the number that is on the scale or the fat cells on our bodies. It should be based on our character and who we are as people. It all starts with how we feel about ourselves. If we feel as though our worth or value is in the hands of others we will always be less than we truly are. We have to love ourselves first and foremost. Once we begin to truly love and accept ourselves we can then do the same for others. I believe this is why I now am able to look other people directly in their eyes and see them. I accept myself and I value who I am and now I have the confidence to show the world who I am and no longer hide.

Chapter 26 - Validation

Blog titled **"I wish I could describe it"**
January 27, 2016

I
t has been nine weeks and three days since my surgery. I cannot believe how much my life has changed in such a short time. I am now down 30 pounds since my surgery date. I have gotten rid of so many clothes. I have gone from a 3XL to a XL/L depending on the fit. I have gone from a size 24W to a 16/18. It is so crazy. I feel more confident and proud. I take time to look nice, instead of just throwing on what fits. I actually get to choose the style and color I like now inside of taking what I can get. I have more energy and excitement for life. Physically, the things that I have noticed since surgery are the feelings associated with eating. For instance, eating too fast makes me sneeze. I know, weird right? It also hurts my stomach and throat if I eat too fast or too much at one time. And it will let

you know within seconds that that was one too many bites. I used to live for sugar, the sweeter the better. Now anything too sweet and I cannot stand it. I also used to love spicy (but not too spicy) food and anything BBQ and now I can major heartburn if I have anything like that. Water, which is a very important part of the weight loss is so hard for me to digest now. It is like liquid cement. And it is not just swallowing it, it is digesting it. It hurts in my stomach and my throat. I have tried all different temperatures to see if I can find something that will work for me, and nothing. I have tried Crystal lite, too sweet. I have tried lemon, not bad. I have to make sure to consume enough water throughout the day, somehow… It kind of sucks but I will take a bit of discomfort in place of all the great things that are happening any day.

Some of the new things that I am finding with my body that are totally awesome are: 1.) I can cross my legs, not perfectly but they are crossed. Something I have never been able to do. Very exciting! 2.) I can reach my arm around my back and scratch my back. 3.) There is so much space between me and the steering wheel I feel like someone should be sitting on my lap. I used to be right up to it with the seat all the way to the back. 4.) All chairs are finally comfortable for me, even movie theatre chairs. I actually have space. Booths are no problem. The real test will be folding chairs in the summer. They were my nightmare. I no longer worry about breaking anything anymore. It is so nice not to have to think about that.

All of those things are so wonderful but there is something that is even better than all of those combined and that is... I FEEL LIKE PEOPLE SEE ME NOW! I am no longer invisible. This is huge, really huge. The world that I have been living in but never really LIVED in is finally acknowledging me. Men hold doors for me and smile at me. Woman don't roll their eyes and make snide remarks to me anymore. Children no longer stare and say Fat or Pregnant. I am seen by people, noticed as another human being and not a problem that needs fixing. All the time that I was overweight I never realized how much it hurt me to be invisible until now. It hurts me to recognize the same pain in others and I wish they knew what the other side felt like. I wish they knew that it could be better and that they didn't have to feel that indescribable pain anymore.

It is so true what they say that you get what you give. I leave my home now feeling confident, comfortable in my clothes and proud of who I am becoming and what I get back is people who see that in me. Acknowledgment and validation from people who too have confidence, are comfortable with themselves and proud of who they are. Recently at the store, my husband looked right past me because he was looking for the old me, the obese woman with her head hung low. The new me is the woman who holds her head high and smiles at those around her just waiting for what comes next. I wish I could adequately describe these feelings that I am having now versus the feelings I used to have. I will simply say this it is like I have gone from static black and white television to HD Technicolor in 3D. Life is better, people are better, the world is better and I feel a heck of a lot better. Two months out and I would never go back. Thank you VSG (vertical sleeve gastrostomy) and Dr. Amson for this gift.

"If you change nothing, nothing will change"

Validation is the one thing that each person in this world needs. To have someone say to us, yes you are right, we understand how you are feeling. Validating someone and their feelings is a true sign of love. Love is as important to each human being as breathing is.

My whole life I searched the ends of the earth looking for this feeling, the words of "You are normal and everything is ok." I never found it. I thought I might find it in food. I thought a pet, or shopping or anything could give it to me. And yet I still never found what I was looking for.

The one person that I wanted and needed it from more than anything was my mother and sadly she could not give it to me either because she did not have the tools to do so. She was unable to give it to herself and so she was not able to give it to me either. If you do not have it to give it to someone, you can't give it. We are taught that validation should come from someone else. But what we should really know is that validation first needs to come from ourselves. When we say to ourselves, "Alicia, you are normal and you are ok and I understand," we then validate ourselves. We give to ourselves what we think we need from others. We become the most important person to ourselves which then reminds us how much we need a good relationship with our number one person, you.

We will treat ourselves with a higher respect and more kindness when we realize we only need to count on ourselves and soon validation from other becomes eliminated as it is no longer important to us the way that our own validation is. Our confidence begins to grow as we learn that we are responsible for our own feelings and no longer rely on the opinions of others to validate who we are or how we feel about ourselves. The bottom line is when we become our own source of validation, we help our confidence begin to grow.

Chapter 27 - Finally ME

Blog titled **"If you would have told me"**
July 2016

My life has changed so much in the last few months; sometimes I look around in amazement and wonder if I'm in the middle of a really good dream that I hope no one wakes me up from. If you would have told me that one day I could walk into any store and pick out anything I wanted in a size medium/large, I would have said you're crazy. If you would have told me that one day I would be one of those woman that men actually take the time to "check out" I would have said, "Quit playing." If you would have told me that one day I'd actually be that woman that other women get angry with because their man actually took the time to check me out, I would have said, "Where are the hidden cameras, am I being punked?" If you would have told me that one day I would be able to keep up physically with my family playing at the park and swimming, I would have said, "This is my dream come true." Lastly, if you have told me that one day I would wake up from this nightmare that used to be my life and now be able to enjoy every moment and experience as the woman I was meant to be HAPPY, I would have to say Thank You!

I cannot even begin to explain how much my life has changed so I will start with the facts.

Fact: 1.) I used to weigh 321 pounds.

Fact: 2.) I now weigh 189 pounds.

Fact: 3.) I only have 39 pounds to go to reach my goal weight.

Fact: 4.) I have lost 132 pounds in total.

Fact: 5. I have lost 70 pounds since the day of my surgery (plus 32 pounds that I lost on my 30-day liquid diet) in 9 months.

And the final and most important of all these facts is that I have never been happier. The weight that I have lost is not the reason that I am happy. It is so much more than that. I am happy because this is the life that I have always wanted for myself. I'm happy because I get have experiences that I have never had before. I am happy because I have confidence and it feels awesome. I am happy because my whole world used to be about how others see me and what they think about me and now finally I could care less what anyone thinks about me. You sure waste a lot of time on caring what others think about you and their opinions. Now my time is spent thinking about the things that do matter such as how can I share my joy with others? How can I be a better Mom, wife, daughter, child care provider and person? Not oh I wonder what that stranger thinks about me? Who cares? They don't matter. The only people that matter are the people that know you and care about you.

When I think back to what a day in my life used to be it makes me sad and grateful. Sad because it took me so long to realize this is not the life that I deserve and grateful because of the life I have now. I had to go through those hard experiences and moments to truly appreciate the life I am now blessed enough to call my own.

I feel like I used to be walking around in a costume with a face that looked like me and a body that looked like me but I was never really myself. My costume looked like me but it was heavy, dark, sad and carried tons of lost dreams with it. Now that I have unzipped this costume to reveal the true me I am light, happy and I carry with me my new found desires and hopes for the future.

So, now I need to share even more of my experiences with anyone and everyone out there.

"Don't stop until you are proud"

This book is more than a how I lost weight from having surgery. This book is a road map to how I have taken this journey from morbidly obese to feeling like I am Finally Me. There have been twists and turns, detours and construction sites and endless long bumpy roads. Now I have arrived at my destination and it is so much better than I ever could have dreamed up. Each person will have their own experience on their journey and all I can wish for you is that it will be a positive one. It will be just that once we learn to take each day as a new experience and try and appreciate the learning that comes from every moment. There will be many, so be open to them.

There are so many things that I have gotten from this journey and it is much more than just losing weight. When you are sitting in your fat self at the start of this trip to this new life, you are thinking that if only I could lose 50-100 pounds, life would become automatically perfect. But the truth of it is that we think we just want to lose weight but what we truly want is to feel normal, feel accepted and have a life that we see everyone else having.

We want to be able to love who we are and what we look like no matter what.

We want confidence and pride.

We want to feel sexy.

We want to think about anything else in life and not just food.

We want to be able to have emotions, feel emotions and when necessary work through our emotions.

We want to love ourselves unconditionally so we can love others in our lives the same way.

We want a life that nothing holds us back, especially our weight.

We want normal.

What if I told you that if you worked hard, tried to lose some weight on your own, went through all the proper channel, the specialists and surgeons ask of you, worked through some emotional weight gaining issues with a counselor or therapist and was able to have the surgery?

Once you had the surgery you continued to follow what and how you are supposed to eat that you could have all these things and so much more. You could be normal and have confidence, feel self love, have pride in who you are and how you present yourself in this world. You could be sexy you could give unconditional love because you have it yourself to give. And nothing could hold you back from this life that you deserve, especially your weight.

Would you take the chance?

Would you do the work?

I feel so very incredibly blessed to say this is the amazing life that I have now. Each thing I had hoped for myself before I had this surgery has come to reality plus so much more. Things I never expected have now become something that I can appreciate daily. You too can have this as your life if you do these few small things beforehand and become Finally You.

As I sit here and write this last page of my book this is my dream for you, to be able to have everything that you have always wished for yourself and so much more. I want your life to be exactly what you deserve, awe-inspiring. I sit here, Finally Me. Finally, I am the Alicia I always should have been, finally happy, finally confident, finally free and so I thank you. Thank you to my doctor, my surgeon, my specialists, my husband, my family, my children, the nurses, friends and strangers who helped along the way. I say thank you to every twist and turn, detour, construction site, endless long bumpy roads.

Last and greatest of all thank you's, goes to myself. Thank you Alicia for choosing you, for choosing this surgery to help get to this amazing life you now have. Thank you Alicia for your hard work, your determination, your sweat and tears. Thank you Alicia for allowing you to become FINALLY ME!

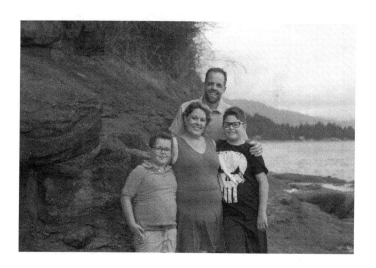

Keep in Touch

If you have found this book to be helpful, I'd love to hear from you. Please take a moment to connect with me on Facebook here:
www.facebook.com/alicia.hillmarceau

Visit my website at: www.marceaubooks.com

My blog: http://peaches150.wordpress.com

Twitter: @ahm2177_alicia

Instagram: @peaches2177

Made in the USA
Middletown, DE
02 August 2017